Reflections along the Way

An Idyll Arbor Personal Health Book

Reflections along the Way

Stories of Recovery and Life

From One Who Has Been There

Barry Bocchieri

Published and Distributed by

Idyll Arbor, Inc.

PO Box 720, Ravensdale, WA 98051 (360) 825-7797

Library of Congress Cataloging-in-Publication Data

Bocchieri, Barry.

Reflections along the way : stories of recovery and life from one who has been there / Barry Bocchieri.

p. cm.

ISBN-13: 978-1-882883-66-0 (alk. paper)

1. Life skills--United States. 2. Conduct of life. 3. Alcoholics--Rehabilitation. I. Title.

HQ2039.U6B63 2007

616.86'103--dc22

2007010919

This one is dedicated to my father and brother – friends, confidants, fellow travelers along the path – and to all those who have come before me in the program who helped me save my life. I owe you a debt I will never fully be able to repay.

Contents

Preface

To all those who have asked for a sequel to my first book, *Things That Work: A No-Nonsense Guide to Recovery from One Who Knows* and who asked for my personal story: Here it is. Although not fully autobiographical; that may come later. This book provides lessons I've picked up along the way in my journey in sobriety and in life.

Like the first book, this one is short, sweet, and to the point. These are things I've learned along the path. Many of them no one taught me, while some were hand-delivered to me on a platter from friends, teachers, and others.

So without further ado, as they say, let us begin.

Acknowledgements

Again for this one I want to thank Patty Shannon, proofreader and typist extraordinaire; to my copy editor, Mindy Reed, thanks for your refinements; and to my publisher, Tom Blaschko, for believing in the project and going forward with it – thanks, Tom.

To the people who have read the manuscript: Lynn Robins, thanks for your detailed feedback; to my father, your late-night hours were greatly appreciated; and to Mae, thinks for your input on the draft.

And again to all the people in twelve-step treatment past and present, who were the real heroes of the book: Thank you all. You saved my life.

1

Sometimes you have to cross the desert – alone

We all have deserts in our life. Everybody has them. Things can be going along fine and then something happens. The death of someone you know, a breakup of a relationship, a divorce, a job loss, bad health. You name it and old Murphy can throw it at you.

I've crossed lots of deserts in my life, just like you have. Or maybe you think that the desert goes on forever. Remember, all deserts have a beginning and an end. Perhaps you're stuck in the old Richard Farina book title: "I've been down so long it looks like up to me."

Well, I'm here to tell you that deserts do end. I've been there, I've crossed them, and I've come back. They always end if you hang in there. You might say, "Well, that's easy for you to say. My brother's dying. Where is the end of his desert?" And that's true for him – that would be, as they say, his final desert crossing. We all make that last crossing alone one day.

But for the rest of us, it's like the heroine says to Indiana Jones in one of his movies: "Indy, fortune and glory are going to get you killed." He responds, "Maybe, but not today." Well, not today for you and not for me, not yet. And in between the "not yet," we can do a heck of a lot, you and I. We could cross the whole Sahara if we had to, assuming we had enough water and supplies, and knew where the waterholes were.

So where are your supplies – your waterholes, so to speak, your points of nourishment and rest along the way? What motivates you to cross the desert? Like the sorcerer asked Conan in the movie, "Tell me the dream in your deepest heart." To which Conan replied, "Valeria," his love, who had died and gone to Valhalla.

What is the dream in your deepest heart? That's what will carry you though. "I don't have one," you say. We all do. You know that's true. Maybe yours is just to survive. There's no shame in that. Why, I'm the best survivor you'll ever know. I've survived more damn things than I care to remember, and you can, too.

Buckle down, saddle your horse, fill your canteens. Get the people, places, and things that will support you on your journey, because you are the only one who can make the journey. But you can't do it alone. You need help – a friend, a sponsor, a meeting, a book, a song, a workout, whatever it is. These are the things you either put in your saddlebag or know where to find them along the way, according to your map of the desert. These will help you get across. And remember: all deserts can be crossed. Safe journey to you.

2
Lighten the load if you are to make the journey

All kinds of things can weigh you down: cars, trucks, houses, relationships, jobs – things. If you're going to make the journey successfully, you have to lighten the load.

I often have my clients, with whom I work (recovering addicts and others), pretend they're flying a large propeller-driven cargo ship, making a transatlantic flight. I tell them to suddenly realize that they don't have enough fuel to make it. I advise them, just as I'm advising you now, to tell your crew to throw everything out that you don't need. Out goes the luggage, out go the seats that you have ripped up. When the crew comes back to you and says, "We threw everything out but the priceless grand piano," you say, "We don't have enough fuel. The piano has to go." They say, "It's priceless." You say, "The piano goes or we all go." They get the point. The cargo door is opened and they push the piano out. This gives you barely enough fuel to make the crossing, but you can now land safely.

In sobriety, we tell people: no major changes for the first year. When you get bogged down in life, you make it harder to accomplish things. In sobriety, it can mean a relapse. In life, it can mean big-time frustration and pain. I see so many people these days trying to do everything. Their plans crash. You cannot do everything. Life requires sacrifices.

For me, the first few years of sobriety were work and meetings. But limiting myself was the best thing I ever did, because it taught me discipline and to trust myself one day at a time. I didn't get bogged down in extra things, things that I didn't need for my journey, the journey of sobriety.

And if your journey isn't sobriety, what then is it? To raise a family, to get a better job, to take up an exercise routine? Whatever it is, remember to lighten the load.

3
When betrayal happens, don't let it make you bitter

Sooner or later (for many people it's sooner), someone or something you know will betray you. It may be real or imagined, but either way, the effect will be the same: emotional shut-down and lack of trust. The walls come up and your world shrinks down and you don't trust. A piece of you becomes deadened and you retreat into your shell.

I've faced my own forms of betrayal in my life. When I was younger, it almost did me in, and I drank and did drugs. When I was older and in recovery, I didn't drink but it almost did me in again – almost.

When this happens, it's okay to pull the wagons in a circle for a while. Take time to reflect and wonder about who and what you are as a person. You can crawl into your cave. But when the dust settles and your wounds are starting to heal, then, my friend, it's time to go back out again. Reconnect with people, go back to those meetings that you have been staying away from, call that old relative that you haven't seen for some time.

And while you're at it (and I know this one isn't easy), try to see it from the other guy's side. This doesn't mean you have to be a doormat or even excuse the behavior as okay. You're only trying to learn from it, to take off the rose-colored glasses and see the world for what it really is – the good, the bad, and the ugly, as they say.

For when you look at it, as I have and do, you will find that it wasn't even betrayal at all, just people doing stupid things, and you got caught in the crossfire, so to speak. It still hurts like hell, but looking at it this way takes a lot of the bitterness out of it and gives you the opportunity to trust again. This time with the rose-colored glasses off and looking at life as it really is. It's not so bad this way, you know. Only different.

4
Break bread with people you care about

It seems we live in a world that, for many of us, is getting more and more out of control. We work long hours, we are increasingly under stress to get things done, and it seems we are all under time constraints of one form or another. As a result of this, we have become isolated. Very few of us break bread with people we care about anymore. We are all too busy.

When I'm counseling people with weight problems, the first thing I tell them is to cook dinner for themselves and invite someone over to share it with them. Oftentimes they look at me like I'm from Mars. When someone has depression problems, I tell them to do the same thing.

I was raised in a twelve-step tradition of "diner therapy." What that means is that there is a meeting in the car before the meeting. You pick someone up in your car or he picks you up and then you go to a diner for coffee or something to eat after the meeting. The purpose is to share with other people, to break the isolation that all addicts feel.

Similarly, when you are home and you cook for yourself (and it can be real simple), you increase the sense of control you have in your life. There are very few things that we have control over, so when we cook for ourselves we exercise control, however small, over what we do.

The Zen people have a saying: A friend is someone who you have to see eyeball to eyeball.

Most of the rehab programs require patients to eat together. It's the same concept. While you're at it, you can pay attention to what you eat. Try to improve the nutritional content of the foods you eat. I've done this over the years and it not only improved how I looked and felt, but also gave me a new added interest and pleasure.

There have been many times in my life when things were going badly, when the only thing I had going right for myself was the fact that I sat down and ate with someone I cared about. Friend, relative, it doesn't matter, just so you don't eat alone. In twelve-step treatment, we say, "I have to go to a meeting if I'm feeling bad." Well, you can bring the meeting into your house by breaking bread with someone, and share a sense of closeness that has been going on as long as people have been on the planet.

5
You don't always have to be comfortable to get things done

I can't tell you how many times one of the people I'm helping comes to me with an article or a book with statements like, "to have real self-confidence in dating, you have to already be dating." Or "to have real self-confidence in the business world, you have to already have a job when you are looking for your next job." These articles suggest that you have to make yourself comfortable first. In short, you have to be comfortable in order to get comfortable. Comfortable – as if no one was ever uncomfortable in their lives.

Some of these people show me Maslow's* "hierarchy of

*Abraham Maslow, for those of you who don't know, was a psychologist who came up with what he called his "hierarchy of needs." On it he put food, water, air, clothing, shelter, sex, and love, in order of importance. Maslow said you have to get one need met first before you can move up to the next higher one.

needs," and they see "sex," so they say, "Love is a need. I have to have my girlfriend [or boyfriend] to feel comfortable." Well, Albert Ellis, the famous cognitive therapist, says love is not a need; it is a deeply held desire from childhood. You will be happier with it, but you can be happy without it. You see, we (especially alcoholics) are not used to seeing things in terms of gradualness. We think in either/or terms.

The point is, if you are, or I am, a little uncomfortable, so what? Did you know that much of the world's great writings were done in prison? So much for being comfortable. In twelve-step treatment we are "big on stabilizing," as the cognitive therapists say. Twelve-step people say, "getting sober." It's the same thing, folks, and follow me on this: Confidence comes from within. Let me say that again: Confidence – true self-confidence – comes from the inside out, not from your girlfriend/boyfriend, husband/wife, job, house, etc. The old saying of "work on you and it gets better," is as important now as it ever was.

Let me tell you a little story to drive home my point.

Now, not to sound too egg-headed on anyone here, but did you know that in the twelfth century, under, I believe, Genghis Khan's grandson, 40,000 Mongol horsemen traveled 6,000 miles? Think of that for a second. That is traveling by horseback from New York to California and back again. And they did it in the dead of the Siberian winter. When they arrived at Moscow, 40,000 of them defeated 100,000 Russian troops.

The Mongolian soldier would sleep on his horse. In times of stress on a long march, they would cut a vein of the horse and drink his blood. Steak tartare came from the Mongolians: raw meat was put under the saddle, and the pounding of the saddle and the sweat of the horse would tenderize the meat.

Genghis Khan was the greatest conqueror the world has ever seen (largest land mass controlled, larger than Alexander the Great). Now, this is more than just a history lesson. And yes, I know the Mongols were "bad dudes," as my young friends say. But here is the point. They accomplished these things and they weren't comfortable when they did them. They were considerably uncomfortable.

Being comfortable is a modern Western psychology tradition. You can get the job done without it. Why, if everybody had to be comfortable, no one would ever sober up. The first year of my sobriety, I was so tense coming off prescription drugs, alcohol, and pot that I didn't sleep much. You know what? It didn't kill me and it won't kill you. And in the end, like old Nietzsche says, "What doesn't kill you makes you stronger."

6
Always have someone you can talk to whom you can trust

Two important words here: "talk" and "trust." Let's break them down one at a time.

Addiction – food, alcohol, drugs, gambling, you name it – each is, basically, a disease of isolation. In fact, I'll go so far as to say that addiction *is* isolation. Or, put another way: without isolation, there can be no addiction. Twelve-step people are really big on this. End the isolation by going to meetings, get with other people and see what happens. The thing is, you need to talk to some people from time to time on a regular basis. This is personal, private time alone. And that comes to the second part of this: trust, my friend. You have got to find someone you can trust. And trust doesn't come easy, and it's not always something you can find right away. It takes time. But find it you must if you're going to survive, because when the winds of adversity blow, I guarantee you're going to need it. For some of you it will be your spouse. For some it will be your sponsor. For others, maybe for now you pay for it, as in a therapist. The point is, you have to find someone who fits the bill. The best ones are free, by the way – friends.

When the stuff hits the fan, as they say, you will be glad that you have someone you can talk to. I've had many times in my life when I was going through a rough time and I was glad there was someone around to talk to.

I can isolate at the drop of a hat. It's easy for me to do and it is even easier in today's world where everyone is more isolated than ever before. It's very easy to get cut off from the mainstream of life.

So find someone you can trust and who is available to talk to you. Very important. I have met many people over time who said they wanted to be my friend, but when push came to shove they simply were not available, or it was too hard for me to get ahold of them. They don't count. The person you choose has to be close at hand. Remember what Don Corleone in *The Godfather* told his family: Keep your friends close and your enemies closer. Well, for now, forget the enemy part – but remember when times get tough and you have to dig in tight, keep your friends close by till the storm passes. You'll be glad you did.

7

It's okay to get scared; just don't stay scared

Facing fear for anyone is not an easy task. Facing fear for someone in recovery, who has used alcohol or drugs to block fear, can be even more overwhelming. There are no longer any chemicals to stop the fear, just you and reality.

In the book *Alcoholics Anonymous*, they use the saying, "living life on life's terms." Well, what does that mean? It means we face life head-on, accepting it for what it is. By accepting it, in time, we transcend it. Not all the time, but enough to fall into what I call the 51/49 rule. If your life is comfortable 51 percent of the time and not comfortable 49 percent of the time, then your life will be worth living.

Sometimes life can seem overwhelming to us. You have a job reversal and are out of work, or you are rejected by someone you care about, or someone who you thought you could trust betrayed you, and now you climb into your shell. You don't go out, you don't call anyone, you isolate. Why?

Because you have been wounded, and as a result, you shut down. Life has given you a low blow. To put it simply, you are afraid.

Well, I'm here to tell you, my friend, it's okay to be afraid. I'm not one of those writers who will tell you things like, "never be afraid." That is ridiculous. We all get afraid and we all – all of us – lose some or most of our confidence from time to time. You know what? Confidence returns if we don't drink, and if we face what it is we fear. If you've been thrown, get back up on the horse, as the saying goes, and stay in the saddle. See how long you can stay on the bucking horse this time before you get thrown off. Maybe you will get thrown off again, but you know what? If you keep getting back up, eventually you will stay on.

Once, when I was sober a couple of years, I was working in the mailroom of an insurance company. Something got me scared – I don't remember what it was now, but it was something. I was living in this garden complex at the time. There were a few recovery people who lived in the complex with me. One of them was Mick. Mick had been a diamond cutter in New York City, a highly skilled trade, I'm told. In the end, he was tending bar in a dive in New Brunswick. On top of this, he weighed all of 130 pounds soaking wet, and he had emphysema, and he smoked. And when he would get annoyed with me, he would yell at me, "Let it happen, you flaky ----" But you know what? I loved this man, because despite his small stature, he had the heart of a lion. Despite his sick condition, I never once heard him complain about himself.

Well, that night, the night I was freaking out, I walked across the courtyard to see him. He lived in a small efficiency apartment, one small room and a tiny, tiny kitchen. I told him that I was planning on taking off from work the next day because I didn't feel well. I didn't exactly tell him that I was afraid, but he surmised. I was sitting on the chair and he was lying on his couch/bed. He said to me, "Why don't you try to go to work?" I mumbled something about not feeling well.

Then he said, "Listen, Barry, you don't know if you can do something until you try."

I looked up at him from where I was sitting. I didn't say anything.

"If you don't like it, you can always leave. But you don't know until you try."

There was such love that went through my veins for that man when he said this, that it stopped me cold in my tracks. It would take me years later to find out what the feeling was, but I felt it nonetheless.

You want the short version of the story?

I went to work, faced my fear, and reached a new level of growth and self-confidence within myself.

Now you say to me, "Well, that's okay for you, Barry. You've had all the recovery people, colorful characters, who were able to motivate you to do these extraordinary things. Well, what about me? I don't have anybody like that."

You know what? I've thought about that for a long time now, and you know what I concluded? You do.

Yeah?

You know why I say that? It's because of this: We all have a little bit of Mick inside us. That's right, all of us. And when you listen close inside of you, you can hear him. Why, he might even be telling you what he told me: "Face your fear. You don't know till you give it a try."

8
Keep your body strong for the journey ahead

There's a lot of territory to cover from the beginning of your journey until the end. How strong are you for the journey ahead?

Your body is all you've got. You know that if it gives out on you somewhere along the way, you're finished. We need strong people for the journey, you and I. Let me ask again: How strong are you?

As we say in recovery, it's mental, physical, and spiritual. People in recovery pay a lot of attention to the mental and a lot to the spiritual, but not much to the physical. In fact, most of them are in denial about it. But the fact is, the physical shape you are in determines to a large extent how effective you are going to be in sobriety.

Why?

Because all we really have is energy. That's it. No energy, no progress. Let me give you an example. Depression is lack of energy. Now, I'm not talking about the suicidal/homicidal, "put me up on the psych ward" type of depression. I'm talking about your general low-level "I don't feel like doing anything, what's the use" depression. In the old days, we would call it the blues or feeling sad or feeling down. Now we call it depression.

You know what helps depression? Exercise.

That's right. Exercise.

We already talked about the power of cooking for depression. Now I'm telling you one more – exercise. And I recommend hard exercise: balls-to-the-wall, break-a-sweat, take-no-prisoners exercise. Now, you may not start out that way. Why, some of my clients start out walking, and that's good.

I work for a major hospital full time; that's my day job. When the patients come through the substance abuse unit there, they are assigned to go to the gym five times a week if they are physically able. You ought to see the changes it makes in these guys in only twenty-one days. And I'm not only talking about how they look. I'm also talking about how they feel and how they think. Remember, as we said, it's mental, physical, and spiritual. Think of it as all three being interconnected and each one affecting the others.

Now, what type of exercise should you do? Well, that's up to you. I recommend lifting weights. That's what I do and I've done it for a number of years now. And if you do it sensibly, over time it will have the most profound effect on you in every area of your life – mental, physical, and, yes, spiritual.

You see, there is something I forgot to tell you. I left the best for last.

Exercise is an inner journey.

That's right. The person you are when you start your exercise program will be very different from the person you will be after you've done it for a while.

Remember when we started this little talk, I asked you how strong you were for the journey. Well, I didn't tell you that the journey of exercise is largely – not only, but largely – an inner journey. And yes, you reap all kinds of other benefits: increased energy, stronger body, improved health. But the true thing you have to overcome in the gym or on the track is yourself. Like the saying goes, "That which lies before me and that which lies behind me is not as great as that which lies within me."

Good luck.

9
All leaders are readers

"What's this?" you say. "Leaders, corporate heads, military generals? I'm not interested in that. I only want to improve my life a little." Well, this rule does apply to corporate types, but it also applies to people who want to lead their own lives.

This is the mental part of the equation that we talked about earlier, and it too has had a profound effect on my life. Through books you can be exposed to ideas that can literally change the course of your life. It's happened to me and it can happen to you. One of the benefits of being a writer is that people come up to you and tell you things, nice things about the way your book touched them. Sometimes a book can speak to you. It can talk to you directly and tell you what you need to know to help you solve a problem in your life.

What kind of books do I recommend? All kinds, but mostly books that will teach you things. Fiction is okay, but don't read just fiction. And don't worry about what other people think about what you read. The main point is to let books help you improve the quality of your life. As the Good Book says, "By the fruits ye shall know them."

Keep a stack of books with you at all times and pick a period of time when you will read, even if it's only a page or two. It adds up, and before you know it, you've finished one more book. And you've learned one more thing and spoken to one more person through the book. And if you're lucky, like I have been, you will meet a few of them and they in turn will change you even more.

Let me talk a little bit about remedial reading – reading you do to help yourself in some area. We have a bit of snobbery in America about reading outside of school. It's like we believe all you need to know you read/learned in school. Anything that has an instructional nature to it, as in teaching you how to do something, is considered taboo. Many people think there is something wrong with you if you read a how-to book. I have a joke about this subject. The second most messed-up people in the world are people who read self-help books. And the most messed-up people are people who never read them.

The way I view self-help books is like this: Many of them are filled with fluff, but if you read them with an eye for picking out one or two or three key ideas, over time you can learn something. I'm not going to get into the whole point of if it is scientifically accurate or not. You decide that. And the way I suggest you do that is to see if it improves the quality of your life. No improvement, no more books by that author. Some or medium or big improvement – then consider what else the author has to say. It's a simple rule and it's worked for me, and I believe it will work for you. Happy reading.

10
Learn that life is mostly an inside job

You've heard this one before too: Life is mostly an inside job. Well, what exactly does that mean? Does it mean that outside events don't bother you? Well, no, I don't think it means that. Remember, I said *mostly* an inside job. It doesn't say *entirely*. If you're hungry, if you're tired, if you're cold or hot, these things will affect you. If you're sick, these things will affect you. If someone dies, these things will also affect you.

But here's the point: We humans over-react and over-generalize. There is nowhere where this is more apparent than in twelve-step recovery – Alcoholics Anonymous, Narcotics Anonymous, Gamblers Anonymous, and Overeaters Anonymous, to name a few.

People come into their first meetings with their lives largely or completely out of control. Their marriage is on the rocks. They have lost their jobs, or they don't have jobs. In short, they are in complete disrepair. And yet people get better and they experience peace and a certain amount of contentment, despite their lives not working and things still being out of control.

Why?

Because people's attitudes about their problems change, not the problems themselves. So here is the proposition for you. If things make you happy, then how come these people in recovery who I am talking about – and I have seen hundreds and hundreds, maybe even thousands over the years – aren't miserable? Because *things* don't make you happy. *You* make you happy. Or, as we started this little section, life is largely an inside job. Your reaction to things is far more important than the things themselves.

In our consumer-driven society, we are told "Buy this and you will be happy," "Buy that and you will be happy, have more sex, be more popular." Or the big one: "Be famous and you will be happy." Or better still: "Be rich and be famous, and you will be really happy." Well, do you think this is true? I think you will be more comfortable. You will have more advantages. But happy? I don't know. Content with yourself? I don't know.

I like the quote by the economist John Kenneth Galbraith. He said something like this: The difference between a little bit and a lot is a great deal, but the difference between a great deal and enough is very little.

The fact that life is largely an inside job has been known throughout the ages. Jesus talked about it; the Buddha talked about it. All the major religions and philosophies talked about it. Some of the easiest times in my life were in early recovery when I had nothing and I was the most content. So remember, life is largely an inside job.

11

Always keep your sense of fellowship, for it is the thing of life

Everybody needs something to believe in, to feel a part of, to belong to. Those who have it are blessed. Those who don't have it don't know what they are missing. In this area, I think the twelve-step people have a bit of an edge. If they're lucky, they get this one down and it saves their lives. That's the lucky ones. The others are not so lucky. Well, you get my drift.

When you belong to something greater than yourself, then your life takes on a whole new meaning and purpose. You have something to look forward to every day.

"What is a fellowship?" you say. I would define it as a group of people who get together for a common purpose, whatever that purpose may be. It could be to stop drinking, to stop over-eating. It could be a group of people who get together to build cars, read, ride bikes, whatever it is. In one of the traditions of Alcoholics Anonymous, it's said that our common welfare should come first. "Personal recovery depends on AA unity." What this means is that, as Benjamin Franklin said concerning the British, "We must indeed all hang together, or most assuredly we will all hang separately." Nowhere is this more apparent than in AA.

Can you have this sense of fellowship with your family only? Yes, but I don't think it is the same thing. When people are brought together for a common purpose, there is a certain – call it what you will – magic, chemistry, vibes that exist nowhere else.

If you go to a twelve-step meeting, you will see a group of rag-tag people who individually don't look like they would have enough sense to come in out of the rain. That is individually. But when these rag-tag people get together to form a meeting, then very positive things begin to happen.

There is a synergistic reaction that takes place. The whole becomes greater than the sum of its parts. A whole group of people who couldn't do anything on their own can, as a group, get sober and help others to get sober, too. And when you feel this feeling, this sense of belonging, it can change your life forever.

I can remember when I first started experiencing this feeling early on in my recovery. I would come to meetings at night and I would have these deep feelings for the other guys at the meetings – strong, powerful, spiritual feelings. Today you would call it bonding. Then, it was a sense of fellowship. There are also other words to describe it: sisterhood, brotherhood, group, fraternity, congregation. You get the picture. It doesn't matter what word you use, as long as you get the meaning.

If I could have one wish for you, it would be this: that you find a fellowship and join it. It will make your life so much richer, and for some of us it will even save our lives.

12
Always have your Higher Power, even though it may change

This is a controversial one. In twelve-step treatment, people who join are encouraged to have a concept of a Higher Power. A Higher Power is defined as anything other than yourself that you can draw on for support and guidance.

"This is religion," you say. Well, yes and no. Yes, if you have a spiritual God; no, if you pick something else. My first sponsor was an atheist. I used to say, "What do you turn it over to, if not a spiritual entity?" He would say, "I turn it over to the trees, the sky." Trusting nature will work if you let it. In the religions of the East (Taoism and Buddhism), nature is a very big part of their religion. Much of their religion is more like a philosophy than a religion. Letting go and following the Tao (pronounced "dow") is close to what twelve-step people call their third step: turning our life and will over to God, as we understand him. You, me, anyone can experience the benefits without believing. Just let go of all the complex questions, like if I was in prison and let go to my Higher Power, would I still stay in prison? Use it in simple matters first and watch your faith grow.

I've known several people over the years who called themselves atheists, and you know what I think? That the atheists have more faith than they think they do. They believe in something: the power of their thoughts. What do you believe in? What gives you order in your life? I know all the arguments that atheists use. I know God can't be proven or disproven. I just have two words for these people: eternity and infinity. That's all, just two very short words that are the deepest words you will ever think about. Eternity: no beginning and no end. Infinity: it goes on forever. This is what the universe is.

"Okay," you say, "what about the Big Bang?" And I say, "What was before the Big Bang?" Now, don't think too long on these things because you can drive yourself wacky. But seriously, as for me, I've always felt that I was a little primitive – you know, like the old prehistoric man first looking up at the stars. There is a sense of wonder that I feel. I don't have all the answers, and that is okay because I'm not the Higher Power. I don't know exactly what is, but it's not me. I see an order, and for me that's enough. I don't need more than that.

Now, over time my conception of my Higher Power has changed, and that's okay, too. Why, I remember a few years ago I thought, what if this whole universe has an intelligence? You know, maybe it's not God as we know it or think about it, but the universe has its own consciousness. I was pretty pleased with myself, until that night I realized that it is called Taoism and it was discovered over two thousand years ago. After my ego was deflated some, someone reminded me that that's okay, because I was thinking in high-level circles. Very little is new under the sun, folks. Most of the things you and I think about have been thought by someone long ago. But – and here is the point – it doesn't matter, because you are still thinking them up for yourself and re-discovering them.

I think a person's sense of his or her own spirituality is one of the most important things a person can have. And don't worry if it changes over time, because like life, it is ever expanding and growing, and may you continue to grow. Good luck to you on your quest.

13 Everyone's problem is different

"What's this?" you say. "I thought everyone's problem is the same. Now you're telling me they are different. What gives?" Well, to me it goes something like this. Problems, like pain, are subjective. This means what is a problem for you may not be a problem for me. We have already tackled this one. What is a problem is not a problem per se, but the person's perception of the problem.

Let me give you an example. I do a fair amount of public speaking. Most weekends I am off doing a seminar or a workshop. I can't tell you some things that have happened to me as a public speaker. You wouldn't believe it. Now to me, this goes with the turf. But to you or someone else, this might be very upsetting. And you might have something that you are used to that wouldn't bother you but would really upset me. It depends upon the person. Everyone's problems are different and unique to them, depending on their life situations and experience.

Once, when I was in recovery less than a year, I went with Mick to a meeting to Princeton. Now, not that I came from the other side of the tracks exactly, but let me say it like this: where I was raised in Edison, New Jersey, was light-years away from what I experienced going to meetings in Princeton. To me, their lives were managed better drunk than mine was sober. Mick used to go nuts when I used to tell him that, but that was how I felt.

So we go to this noon meeting and this woman I didn't know at the time, who was maybe in her early forties, was complaining about the fact that she was only going to get two thousand dollars alimony when her divorce went through. Now to me, two thousand dollars a month – and this was back in the eighties – was like a million dollars. If memory serves me correctly, I wasn't working at the time and had trouble making rent. After the meeting I started complaining to Mick. "Who does she think she is? Why, if I had two thousand dollars..." that sort of thing.

He said to me, "Dummy." (He always had a nice way of talking to me.) "To her, her problem of two thousand dollars a month is as big a problem as your problem of not making rent. Everybody's problems are different. They are unique to them."

You know, I never forgot that. All these years later, I can still hear him saying that to me.

We have an old saying in recovery. It's probably not unique to recovery, but that's the first place I heard it. It goes like this: If you put everybody's problems in a room and everybody had a chance of picking up whatever problem they wanted, most people would wind up picking up their own.

As they say, "the grass is always greener, except when it's your grass." So remember, everybody's problems are different, and the guy next to you at the meeting or in life may not be doing any better than you.

14
Sometimes to change something, you do nothing – for a while

A lot of us think that to change something, we have to do it all at once – now. And I understand that a lot of people think this way. I think this way, when I don't catch myself. This is a very Western view. But in the East, in the ancient East, they had a different way of looking at it. Sometimes to change, you do nothing – for a while.

Once when I was in recovery for a couple of years, I went to my sponsor, Carl. I was smoking about two packs of cigarettes a day at the time and I wanted to quit. One of my recovery buddies developed lung cancer and had to have his lung removed. He lived, but it wasn't a pretty sight.

I said, "Carl, I want to quit smoking, but a part of me doesn't want to quit. I don't know what to do."

He said, "Keep smoking. Just accept the fact that for now, a part of you wants to quit and a part of you doesn't. Keep smoking if you want."

"I feel guilty."

"Don't feel guilty. When you're ready, you'll quit."

Now, I know this is not exactly conventional wisdom, but you know what? It worked. And as memory looks back on it, just like Carl said, when I was ready, I did quit. It took me a couple of times, but I eventually made it.

So what is the principle? The principle is acceptance. Or as we call it in twelve-step treatment: surrender. I give up (for the time being) getting what I want, and give in to a power greater than myself. So you don't have a Higher Power? That's okay. Then let what I'm telling you be the Higher Power. Not me, but my words – or Carl's words. Let the message be your guide.

A lot of writers tell you to set goals, that you have to know what you are doing. And that is true for some people. But for many of us, we don't always know which way to go. Many times, for us doing nothing for a while is one way to deal with it. Another way of saying it is, "letting go." Why, you can even "let go" as a life goal. I never set a goal to become a writer. It just came as a result of other things I was doing. I let go, worked on myself, and the rest took care of itself.

So remember: Sometimes to change something, you do nothing – sometimes.

15
Life has a rhythm and a flow to it; catch the rhythm and ride the wave

All of life has a rhythm and a flow to it, and if you listen closely beneath the waves, you can often hear it. And if you look closely beyond the breaking of the surf, you can oftentimes see the rhythm dance in front of you.

I work, as I said, for a major hospital in East Orange, New Jersey. And the rhythm and pace of East Orange is totally different from where I currently live in Edison, New Jersey. Edison is more laid back, more suburban; while East Orange is faster paced, more talkative – one might even say alive. I defy anyone to come for coffee on a Monday morning when you're a little depressed, because you don't want to be there and just see what goes on.

Let me take you through a typical scene. I walk into the main lobby. One of the ex-patients says, "Hey, I relapsed. Can you help me get back in treatment?" Another one wants to tell me that he is now doing well, he is sober, and he thanks me. Another one yells out my name. I look over and wave. Someone over on the other side of the lobby is pushing someone in a wheelchair. I see two of my current patients waiting to take the shuttle bus over to our other hospital to go for a substance abuse screening, and they are nervous. Another one waves to me. And where I work, I might add, is kind of like the United Nations, all races and nationalities all mixed together. And you know what? It makes it interesting, and oftentimes exciting. I defy anyone to stay depressed walking into that scene on a Monday morning.

Suburbia has its own rhythm, much slower, much more subdued. The pace that I described above would be inappropriate in suburbia. And the pace of suburbia would be inappropriate where I work.

As with places, the same can be said of people. Young people have a rhythm, old people have a rhythm. Animals have a rhythm, too. When I go down to the park where I live, I see geese waddling in formation. They have a rhythm. The squirrels that quickly dart back and forth and run up the tree have a rhythm.

Groups have a rhythm, too, which is similar but not the same as places. A twelve-step meeting in suburbia will have a completely different rhythm than a meeting in the city, and so it goes.

Sometimes, through formal structure, the natural flow tends to get beaten out of things. What I mean by that is too much control blocks spontaneity. That's why some of the best meetings I've been to have been "down and dirty" meetings, people just off the street, the kind of people who still see hell in the background. These, for me, are oftentimes the best ones.

Work can have its own rhythm. Spontaneity can be stopped at work by chaos. Chaotic people can break your flow. You can break your own power. I've found that I can do twice as much if I keep centered, out of the way of chaos. (This is not always possible.) When you do this, you develop your own rhythm, and you can accomplish your own flow and your own power. Although it is not effortless, it is much less effort. This to me is what they talk about as Zen-like, being in the flow.

Find the rhythm of the place you are in, then find your own flow in relation to that. That is where your true power lies.

16

Life is not an accounting ledger

Or: how it was doesn't mean that is how it has to be

Many of us go through life thinking that life is some sort of accounting ledger; that just like a ledger, I have to be at this point at this particular time in my life, and if I'm not there, then I'm a failure.

How do I know? Because I lived it. And I've seen other people live it. I've seen hundreds, maybe even thousands of people by now who have turned their lives around after being complete failures.

They hadn't graduated college at age twenty-two, married at age twenty-four, had a house at age twenty-eight, and career advanced at thirty with two children at thirty-two. I'm talking about people who were bottomed out, down and out, over, nothing left – and they came back.

That's how it was for me. At twenty-eight I thought my life was over. I'll be more blunt: For me, my life *was* over. And had I continued going in the direction I was going, I would have been... well, you get the picture. But I found something else that worked for me, and that was twelve-step treatment. When I came in, I was hooked on marijuana, Valium, alcohol, and sleeping pills. Today the rage in suburbia is painkillers. Where I work as a counselor, it's crack and heroin. For some, it's gambling; for others, it's food; for still others, it's loneliness. Whatever it is, they can't make their lives work.

And for these other people, they have found things that worked for them. Maybe it's church, maybe it's sports, maybe the love of a good woman or man. Whatever it is, it is something that when you encounter it, it turns your life around, one step at a time.

Instead of having a corner office with their name on it, these people were looking at a headstone. These people, like me, were looking at the ghosts of past, present, and future, and the future ghost wasn't very pretty. In fact, it said end of the world – death.

So for many of us, we have risen from the dead, been placed back on Earth, enabled to walk among the land of the living one more time – to be free.

The accounting ledger concept is wrong. Wrong for me, wrong for you, wrong for so many of us. The way it was doesn't mean that's the way it has to be. You can change. You can pull yourself out of your mess, turn your life around, and go on.

The journey is the thing, and when you move through the journey and come out the other side, you will, as we say in recovery, experience a new peace and a new happiness. We won't regret the past or choose to close the door on it. The Bible says, "The last shall be first." Maybe the old Good Book was talking to you.

17

Sometimes you just don't take no for an answer

If this seems like a contradiction, then that is because life is a contradiction at times. One of my first mentors in recovery used to say that we should switch the Serenity Prayer around to say, "God, grant me the courage to change the things I can, the serenity to accept the things I cannot change, and the wisdom to know the difference" to put a little more emphasis upon *change*. With an emphasis upon acceptance in twelve-step treatment, you think it strange that I begin this talk with saying sometimes you don't take no for an answer? So what is going on here?

I think there are certain things in your life that are so important to you that you just don't take no for an answer. That means that you go on toward your goal no matter what. There is no turning back. The Romans believed in conquer or die. Caesar said, "The die is cast," when he crossed the Rubicon River. Once he crossed the Rubicon, there would be no turning back.

Conventional wisdom in psychology says that if I can't get what I want and I'm not happy, then there has to be something wrong with me – that an unhappy life is a series of demands. I don't think life is that simple. If someone somewhere hadn't been upset at something and decided he was going to fix it, invent it, explore it, you name it, whatever the "it" is, we may all still be living in caves.

You may ask, "So what you're saying is that we should act like babies if we don't get our way?" Or, "It's the old I want what I want when I want it routine?"

No, I'm not saying that at all. What I am saying is that we – you and I – are much stronger than we think we are. We come from primitive ancestors, who had to bag a prey and drag it back to camp, where we had to survive winter and drought and famine. We still carry the same genes. We are not weak. Yes, society keeps us down and circumstances keep us down and our own beliefs keep us down, but mostly *we*, you and I, keep us down.

So now you're asking, "What if I don't get what I want – the job, house, girl, guy, fill in the blank – what are you saying? It's okay to kill myself, drink, become depressed?" No, the rules of engagement still apply. You work your program, you go to work, you attend to your family. You do what needs to be done, but you don't stop going for what you want. No turning back. It's also called "the code of the warrior." No retreat, no surrender. You face your problem head-on, and if you don't succeed, that's too bad.

When you finally establish this point of view, there is a certain peace that comes over you because now the process is simple. You're not going to quit, no matter what. If you succeed, fine. If you don't succeed, fine too. Either way, you win. You start to realize what the playwright George Bernard Shaw said: "The second greatest tragedy is not getting what you want; the greatest tragedy is getting it." You loosen up and you begin to realize that the journey is the thing. And that through the journey, you've developed something that many people don't have: a code – your own private code of conduct, if you will, for you. But you didn't read it out of a book; you developed it along the way. And you realize that the world isn't a bad place to be, even if you don't get what you want. And you know what? When you reach this point, you might just well get it.

18

The Zen archer

Or: Why you should sometimes go out with only one arrow in your quiver

Conventional wisdom says that when you go out to accomplish something, you should try a lot of times to accomplish what you want. Send out a lot of resumes for a job, ask a lot of girls out for a date, call on a lot of customers if you're a salesman. And there is nothing wrong with this advice. It's called the law of averages, or the numbers game, also called the shotgun approach.

But there is another approach, which in some situations can produce as good or better results. It is the rifle approach. It was, in ancient times, called the Zen archer approach. Unlike the other archers who went out with a full quiver of arrows, the Zen archer went out with only one arrow in his quiver – the purpose of which was to develop focus.

So how is your focus? Do you know what it is that you want to accomplish? The recovery community tends to be fairly small. Everybody knows everybody. A lot of the advice I get from people who are not in recovery does not apply to what I do. I do better focusing on those people who are interested in what I have to say and can identify with me. That doesn't mean I don't try to focus on non-recovering people. It's just that I know my target audience and I know what I do well. I no longer run all around trying to do too many things at once. I develop focus. I know what I want, then I go after it.

The point is that with focus comes clarity. With clarity comes power. So what I'm saying is that sometimes it's not just a question of numbers. Sometimes it's about picking your target well.

Think what it is that you want – that girl, that guy, that job, that sale. Then let the arrow fly. In recovery we have a saying: First things first. This means that the first thing you focus on is your sobriety or your problem, whatever that is. "Do what you can, with what you have, where you are," as Teddy Roosevelt said. The worst of all fears is the fear of living.

So don't let people tell you that it is always a law of numbers. Sometimes it is and sometimes you only need one arrow. You only have one shot, so make it good.

Think deeply about what you want, then go at it one arrow at a time. I'll bet you hit the mark.

19

The corollary to doing nothing

Or: Why sometimes you have to change everything or at least something

"What is this," you say, "another contradiction?" Well, yeah.

"Why?"

Because, as I've said earlier, life is sometimes a contradiction. We have an old saying in recovery. It goes like this: "Give an alcoholic a rut and he'll move in and furnish it for you."

How do you get in a rut?

By not changing anything – for a long time.

That's what addiction is. Some part of you is in a rut. You

have to figure out what it is and change it or accept it.

When I first started counseling, I worked at a beautiful hospital in Red Bank, New Jersey, right on the Navesink River. Sailboats in the summer, ice boats in the winter, millionaires everywhere. I built up a private practice on the side and if I wanted to, I could have stayed there for the rest of my life. But something was pulling at me. "Move on," it seemed to say. "Find out what else is out there." So I made a shift and through a number of zigzag turns I wound up where I am today, working in North Jersey, only some fifteen miles from New York City. I even teach in New York City part time. A whole other world. And for me it's what I needed to do. Along the way I picked up a Master's degree and wrote a book.

Today, my life is so much fuller and richer than it was a few years ago. But my circle of fear has been expanded, and what I mean by that is that when we push the envelope of our comfort zone and confront our fear, the new area that we are comfortable in grows.

In short, your world grows, your circles expand, and your confidence grows in one fell swoop. Well, almost – but you get the idea. So what is your circle of fear? What do you have to do to break out, to come to the other side? What price are you willing to pay for your freedom? I knew what mine was. What's yours?

Maybe it's not a major geographic change that you need. Sometimes small things can make all the difference. If you've been going to the same twelve-step meetings for years, maybe it's time to change up and go to a different one.

How much television are you watching? I've known guys who have taken the TV out of the bedroom and it changed their lives. I've also known people who have stopped watching or have cut way down on their TV watching. Not ready to do any of that? Change the shows you're watching. If you watch crime shows, watch the Discovery Channel. How about how you dress? If you always dress casual, dress up once in a while. If you dress up, dress casual. Your choices are endless. The point is that when you change one thing, you change everything. So get out of that rut: find something to change and do it.

20
It's still a day at a time

Or: Why living a day at a time is the only real way to live

When I first came into the program, they told me I had to, "not drink for one day at a time." That simple little saying saved my life.

Why?

Because not drinking or not drugging forever was too much for me, too overwhelming. You might as well have told me to go to the moon for all the relevance it had for me. But a day at a time I could handle. That is, once I got the hang of it. I never planned to stop drinking. It just happened one day at a time. I never planned on quitting drugs; it just happened one day at a time. I never planned to quit smoking. Well, you get the idea. Breaking things down to bite-size chunks is the only way to go when the project seems too big to handle.

It was years later when I began to study some of the Eastern religions like Zen and Taoism, which stress living in the *now*. I realized that "a day at a time" was the twelve-step way of saying the same thing – a little more concrete, a little more Western, but living in the now nonetheless.

Making a decision in the present is where your real power comes from. That's where you can change things. We have a saying in recovery: "When I have one foot in yesterday and one foot in tomorrow, I'm peeing on the present." It's a little gross but it drives the point home.

Nobody knows what the future holds, despite what various experts claim. There are too many possibilities. Nobody can calculate the odds. When you choose in the present, you let go of the outcome. This is where the first three steps of the twelve steps come in. I can't choose in the future; nobody knows the future. When you let go after your choice, you let go to the great mystery of life. It *is* a mystery, you know, a great adventure, and nobody knows the final outcome. But – and this is a big but – the more choices you make with your eyes open in the present moment, the brighter your future will be. Because every present moment makes up the future.

Now, how you respond to the present moment has been a subject of much debate for centuries. How much are you ruled by the past? How much is present choice? I've read some of the concepts, and a lot of it is a little too deep for me. What I suggest is that you live a day at a time to the best of your ability and let it go at that. The rest will fall into place and you won't have anything to worry about if you do that.

This doesn't mean you don't set goals. Set all the goals you rationally want, just don't forget that no matter what you do, it's always a day at a time. And don't forget where your true power is: right here, right now, not some point off in the distance. Seize your opportunity and act on it, and welcome to a whole new world – a world where you make the choices for you.

21
Armageddon and how I was raised in recovery

Or: Good teachers come in the most unlikely packages

I've had two lives: The life I had with my natural biological parents and the life I had during my early years in recovery. Two different sets of people, both raising me: one conventional, one not. One kind of respectable, at least on the surface, and very middle class. And one kind of rag-tag, not so conventional, kind of rough around the edges.

People often ask me, "Where did you learn your concepts of spirituality from? What professors, philosophers, taught you the things you know?"

My teachers were drunks, former drug addicts.

"Well, what did they do for a living?"

Carpenters, truck drivers, bartenders, convicted felons, prostitutes, bikers, murderers, and a whole assortment of people who just screwed up life. And you know what? They did a pretty good job of teaching me. Don't ask me how they did it. I still don't know, not fully. But they did do a good job. And most of them had very average educations. I might add that they controlled one of the most difficult behaviors to control: alcohol and drug use.

"Well, how did this come about?" you ask.

I think in part it came about because everyone cared for each other. We knew we all had to hang together or the disease would pick us off one at a time.

I came into this world at the age of thirty, fully formed, at least in body. That was the age of my recovery date. Spiritually and emotionally were two different things. You see, I never grew up, not really. My life was put in suspended animation, preserved in a haze of marijuana, amphetamines, alcohol, and tranquilizers. Doomed, or so I thought, to exist this way because that is what it was, just existing. Never to know a dream like other people, to own a house, to raise a family, to have a career. And then, through a series of events (some good, some bad), I found myself in the rooms of recovery. And that is when I was introduced to my first teachers. But not the teachers of the formal classrooms. These were the teachers of the classrooms of recovery. All types of people, a rag-tag group as I said – outcasts, every one. Shunned by society, all of them, in one way or another, even the housewives and the executives.

Losers, cast-off drunks, liars, cheats, failures, you name it and they were it.

And they were good teachers, every one of them. There was God-is-my-sponsor John, although everybody knew your sponsor was supposed to be a person. There was for the rest of my life "I'm an alcoholic, Robert." Everyone knew it was a day-at-a-time program, but it didn't bother these people. They were all eccentric, all a little off one way or another. But they had one thing: They all cared for me. They all helped me and they let me be my own crazy self. And I was plenty crazy back then.

If you've never seen the movie "Armageddon," well, it's my favorite comic-book movie. Bruce Willis stars in it, and it's about these rough-and-tumble blue-collar oil riggers who are called upon by NASA to save the world from this giant asteroid that is on a collision course with earth. Liv Taylor plays Bruce Willis' daughter, and in one scene she is complaining to him because all these guys helped raise her on these oilrigs and she didn't have a normal childhood. Later on in the movie she realizes that they did a fine job.

Well, that was me. The guys who raised me the second time did a damn good job, and they were all characters right out of the movie. So what's my point? You never know who is going to come around to touch you. The things you need to help you, save your life, may come in unconventional packages. Why, you might sit around at a meeting or some other place one day, and someone similar will look over and extend their hand to you and say, "Hi, my name is John" or Robert or whatever, and you'll smile, bite your cheek, extend your hand and say, "Pleased to meet you, my name is..." and you will tell him your name and you will know you've met your new family.

22
Sometimes you know more than you think you know

The Joe McD. story, or how I got out of the mailroom

When I was sober for about two years, I got this job working in the mailroom of an insurance company. It was a job I could have handled with two hands tied behind my back when I was in high school, but because I was newly sober it was giving me trouble.

I had a broken-down car that I used to drive to work, and every other week it seemed it would break down. In the morning one of my tasks was to pick up the mail at the post office. There were usually two big canvas bags, and I would put them in my car and back up to the door at the mailroom entrance of the insurance company and drop them off.

On days when my car would break down, I would take a cab. Sometimes it would cost me more to take the cab than what I earned for the day. But I wanted to get to work and hold onto the job. Also I would have the cab driver stop at the post office and load the mail bags in the cab, then have the cab back up to the insurance company door so I could drop the mail off. Quite a sight, I might add. I never did ask people who worked there what they thought. I can only guess.

The job gave me trouble. You needed to move fast to put all the mail in the slots. I had trouble doing it. The girl I worked with looked like Pamela Anderson and acted like Rosanne Barr, and any time she got mad at me for something I would do, she would complain to my boss and he would always take her side.

I was always complaining about the job at meetings and anywhere else that people would listen to me. It was a constant source of stress to me. One day, my cousin Bart came over to my apartment with Joe McD. Joe was a big African-American guy. To give you an understanding of how big Joe was, my cousin Bart was six-foot-two, two-twenty, and he was small compared to Joe.

So Joe and Bart sat down at my kitchen table. I got them a cup of coffee. In Joe's hands the coffee cup looked like a Chinese teacup. After about a minute of complaining about the mailroom (where I had been for a year at this point), Joe leaned over to me, pounded the table with his huge hand and said, "You got three years of sobriety, you got a college education, you got no business working in the mailroom." The whole room seemed to shake after he said this, and then there was quiet.

Now, Joe was old school, and he didn't care much for alcoholism counselors. But he said to me, "Hell, if somebody's going to do it, it might as well be you."

That is how I make my living today.

Now, the point is I could have changed jobs sooner than I did, but I was new to sobriety and didn't know my way around, so to speak. With McD's size, his personality, his sobriety (he was sober for years at the time), he made an impression on me. The whole gestalt hit me at once and I knew what I had to do.

Here's the point: What do you know about that you're not taking action on? Where is your stuck point? You might not have someone as colorful as Joe McD come into your life, but you know what? We all have a little bit of Joe McD in us – the part of us that is larger than life, a little bit outrageous, a little bit over the top, a character. Inside you or inside someone else, there's a piece of Joe. Listen to them when they talk to you. Listen to yourself when you talk to yourself. Why, they might say something to you that by now you've heard before: "It's time for you to get out of your mailroom."

And when it happens, there will be a little smile on your face and a little twinkle in your eye, and you'll think of me and you'll think of Joe, and you'll know you're on your way up.

23
Silence is not always weakness

Or: How assertion is not always strength

There is a lot of talk these days in recovery circles and elsewhere about telling people what you feel, how it's healthy to tell people what you feel, and all that. My answer to that is sometimes it is and sometimes it's not. You have to consider your goal when you are telling someone what you are feeling or thinking. Albert Ellis, the famous psychologist, tells the story of a young girl in his group, a single mother, who was told by the group to confront her boss in reference to some dissatisfaction she had on the job. The end result was her boss fired her on the spot. Again, think of your goals when you are expressing yourself.

Assertion is not always strength, and silence is not always

weakness. We have had this view in the recovery community for a number of years now, to always tell it like it is. Many times the best solution is just to be quiet. If you can do this, things can oftentimes work out on their own. So if you think about it, in the twelve-step literature there isn't a great emphasis on telling it like it is. There is more of an emphasis on acceptance.

So the tell-it-like-it-is mentality didn't come from the twelve-step recovery literature. "Well then," you ask, "where did it come from?" I think it came from the rehabs, from the great thrust of psychology in America that has been prevalent in the last twenty years.

I can't tell you the number of people I have counseled who have, in addition to losing jobs, have lost relationships and friends, along with having a whole assortment of other ills because they "told someone how they felt."

Now let me clear up a few things. I am in favor of telling the other person how you feel if it is necessary, and then it should be done (if at all possible) calmly and politely. Most of the time, however, it's better to talk to your sponsor, therapist, or another friend, or just reflect on it and think about it before acting. Many times when you say something in a fit of anger, it can't be taken back, especially when you attack someone with your fury. When you're furious with them, it can be disastrous.

Most people don't want to hear the truth from you if it conflicts with their carefully constructed defense mechanism that they use to conceal their inner feelings. Some people will want to hear it, but most don't. The Bible says that the prophet is never recognized in his home country. Truer words were never spoken. At work, where I'm accepted as the teacher, it's a little easier to confront one of the patients – a little. At home or in my personal life, that's another story. Most of the time, they don't want to hear anything. Why? Because I'm not accepted as the teacher there.

Now, I'm not proposing that you be a marshmallow. And I'm not proposing that you don't confront people if you feel you have to. All I am suggesting is that you consider the concept of silence so you can let the true meaning of what I'm saying sink in, which is that assertion is not always strength, and silence is not always weakness.

24

You work on yourself or your self will work on you

This is the one a lot of people have trouble with. They can't understand why they have to work on themselves – their character defects, as we say in twelve-step treatment.

Well, what "self" are we talking about? You have two selves, you know; at least as far as recovery goes. You have your sober self and you have your addictive self. They are both alive and well, living inside you. Who is going to win out in the end will determine who you ultimately will become. You will be either sober or drunk; fat or thin; depressed or relatively happy. Take your pick. You work on yourself or your self will work on you.

We have a saying in recovery that I mentioned earlier that says, "It is recommended that you make no major changes for the first year in recovery." The reason for this is it gives you time to stabilize, to work on yourself one day at a time.

When I sobered up, people did this. Nowadays, with all the emphasis on success and money and relationships, nobody wants to do it anymore. But there is a world of common sense in waiting a year to make changes. We used to say also in recovery (and they still say it, to a certain extent) that, "I don't want to do anything that will make me uncomfortable." Now, this doesn't mean that I never do anything that ever makes me uncomfortable. It means that if it is in violation of my own inner sense of what is right for me, then I don't do it.

After all these years, I still do not like to go into bars. And it's not because I'm tempted, although that is part of it. It's because I don't feel comfortable in the environment, so I don't go. I've got no business being there normally. And in early sobriety, it was years before I ever went into a bar. Now, this is not a lecture on drinking. It is more to the point of trying to tell you that we all, I think, have to honor our true self, the self that wants to grow. A lot of times it gets drowned out by all the noise and chaos of modern life.

Someone once asked the previously mentioned psychologist Albert Ellis how many people worked on their self-defeating personality traits. This is the same, I think, as what twelve-step people call character defects. He said maybe ten percent. He went on to say that most people will work on themselves to improve at their job or to get or maintain a relationship, but not just to work on themselves with no other thought than they want to be conscientious people. But he said the rewards are well worth it.

I couldn't agree more. The rewards far outweigh the costs.

We live in a world where internal work is not valued. It is considered too esoteric, too touchy-feely almost. But there is no finer thing you can do for yourself. Like compound interest, the rewards will pay back to you dividends that you dream about. I've gotten in debates with people over the years who had more things going for them than I – better careers, home life, degrees – you get the idea. But I couldn't identify with their particular problems. It took me a long time to realize it was because I had worked on myself and they hadn't. "How do I know?" you ask. Well, I can't prove it. But the one thing that stood out in my mind was that I was in recovery and they weren't.

I knew adversity and they didn't. I'm talking about coming-from-behind adversity, feeling that you are left behind and then coming back.

As the comic strip character Pogo said, "We have met the enemy and he is us." Well, when you meet you on the battlefield of life, my advice for you is let the sober growing self win out over your less mature self. If you do this on a regular basis, the rewards will amaze you.

25
You never know who will help you – the credit story

When I first came around to recovery, my credit was pretty shot. In fact, I couldn't get a loan to buy a quart of milk. Well, not exactly, but you get the idea. My family didn't trust me and my credibility wasn't the best.

Sometime after I got my first counseling job, I knew I needed to buy a new car. The one I was driving was at least fifteen years old. I used to do a lot of speaking at meetings back then, traveling from group to group, telling my story. One of the guys I knew heard me speak and said he knew my father from the old neighborhood. He told me to come down to his dealership and he would see if he could help me out with a used car. I had let it be known to him that I was looking to upgrade.

When I went into the dealership the next day, I asked for this fellow (his name was Bob). Later in his office he said, "I can help you get a loan if you want a car. I have an in with the bank."

"My credit is pretty bad."

"Well, let me see what I can do."

Later, I said, "How did it go?"

"They weren't going to give you the loan. They said, 'He has defaulted on a loan from his own bank [which was true] and he has been late on other payments. If we give him a loan he'll beat us too.' I said, 'He won't beat you for the loan. I'll vouch for him.' So they said, 'Well, okay, if you vouch for him, we'll give him the loan.'"

Later, Bob said to me, "Boy, your credit was pretty bad."

"I told you."

"Well, enjoy the car. I'll see you at the meeting this week."

"Thank you."

And that is how I got my credit back. When you're in recovery, you never know where the help will come from.

I tell the guys I work with, if you look to me for all of it and we have a personal relationship going, you're screwed because I will fail you, because I'm human. But as Bob Earle, a prominent AA speaker, says, "The people (or multitudes of people) will always be provided to you if you avail yourself to the program; and usually from sources where you least expect it."

When I spoke at the meeting, I didn't speak thinking I would get a reward. I just spoke. The rest followed from that. "Do the thing," the saying goes, "and you will have the power." Only in this case, "the thing" was speaking. The power came later, when I got the help with the loan. Or on a deeper level, you can understand what the Buddhists talk about when they say right action follows right livelihood. That when I'm in alignment with my sober purpose, things oftentimes fall into place. And you then can understand the true meaning of "you never know who will help you."

26

Bikers, suits, housewives, and students

Or: How a rag-tag group of people changed the world (well, almost)

When I came into the fellowship, it was a very exciting time. It was before managed care started shutting down all the rehabs. The first phase of the baby boomers, burnt out, were just coming into the program and the old-timers from World War II were still alive and in a leadership role at meetings.

In one of the recovery clubs I used to go to, it was not uncommon to see, at the same meeting, a biker sitting next to a housewife sitting next to a guy in a business suit sitting next to a homeless person, all sharing, all expressing their points of view on recovery. Everyone respectful of everyone else. And believe me, a lot of these people were pretty rough and they all got along.

Now here's the question for you: If this group of people could get along, what's to prevent other people from getting along? The answer is: Nothing. You just have to want it bad enough; that is, everybody must want it. That, and you need a set of unifying principles like the twelve steps and twelve principles that have proven themselves over the test of time. Oh, yeah – you have to believe that if you don't follow the principles, you'll die. I forgot to tell you that.

When you have the combination of things that I just mentioned, then amazing things can happen. You can even change the world. I've seen every faith I know follow the twelve steps – Jews, Muslims, Christians, Hindus – and they all achieved sobriety. I've also seen all sorts of formerly antisocial types, people who have done all sorts of things up to and including murder, get sober. That's not counting people with psychiatric problems, people with physical problems, unemployment, homelessness, things like that. They all got sober.

Well, if they can do it, guess what? Other people can do it, and other people are just the world. The question is, do people want it bad enough, and are they convinced they can't do it their way?

That's the thing. If I think I can do it my way, then I'm not going to try your way. If I think I'm God, then I'm not going to let God be God. We have a saying in recovery, "I can't be God,

I'll let him/her/it do it."

When outcasts get together, they can change the world if they follow the steps. "What's all this talk of changing the world?" you say. Well, let me tell you a little story we used to say in recovery. A little boy goes to his father and says, "Read to me." The father is busy and instead gives the boy a page from a magazine that has the world printed on it. He tears it up and tells the little boy to see if he can put it back together again. He figures this will keep the boy occupied for a while. Instead the boy comes back in a few minutes with the puzzle completed. When the father asks the boy how he completed the puzzle so quickly, the boy says, "It was easy. On the other side of the page was a picture of a man, and when I put the man together, the world fell into place."

So you get the picture: to change the world, you change you. And if all of us change ourselves, guess what can happen? You say you're not that important? Well, think on this for a minute. I want you to think about how Alcoholics Anonymous happened – with two people getting together. Two rather inept people, I might add: an out-of-work stockbroker and a doctor – a proctologist, to be exact – getting together at an opportune moment. And as a result, over a million people owe their lives to them. You are important. Alone we may be weak, but together we are strong. Peaceful coexistence is the way to change the world one day at a time, through you.

27
Street people, drug addicts, and winos

Or: How I learned to identify, not compare

I got sober in a storefront operation called "The Open House" in New Brunswick. A storefront operation, for those of you who don't know, is just that: a store or a building that is rented, usually in a bad neighborhood, that helps people recover.

When I came to the Open House, I was a middle-class kid from suburbia exposed to street hustlers, heroin addicts, and homeless people. Most of the people I sobered up with were minority people, blacks and Hispanics. In fact, in many of my first group therapy sessions, I was the only white person. What I noticed was how caring everyone was for me, despite our differences. I wasn't sure I could identify at first. But I found that people who came from deprived backgrounds often had a richness to their descriptions of their experience that was unlike anything I had heard before.

My first sponsor when I finally got clean of everything was a black man by the name of Rufus. Rufus was sober ten years when I met him. I was so overwhelmed by the prospect of going completely cold turkey, off all the stuff I was on, that I told him once I didn't think I could stay sober even one day at a time.

He told me his story. He, at the time, had been a counselor for ten years at the Open House.

"At the end of my drinking, I was a bum. Kicked out of my house, nowhere to go. I woke up in the park and all I wanted was my next bottle of wine. Somewhere inside me I said a prayer. I asked God to help me. And it was the darnedest thing. I swear it was as if this beam of light came down and showed me a path to the first meeting I went to. If I live to be a hundred, I'll never forget it.

"Later on, I asked God to give me ten years. That's all I wanted, just ten years. I've got ten now, so I guess I can't complain."

You can laugh, folks, but I was raised on those types of stories. And after he shared with me his "experience, strength, and hope," as we say in the rooms, I didn't have any problems of feeling overwhelmed that day or the day after or the day after that. This didn't happen all at once, but gradually, over time, till I *knew* I would make a full recovery.

That was when I first learned what it meant to identify, not compare. As the saying goes, "We are all brothers under the skin." Your pain is my pain, your joy is my joy. Rufus's background was as different as you could get from my middle-class upbringing, but man, could I identify with him. I also came to understand what was meant when they said, "alcoholism and addiction are equal opportunity diseases." They don't care what your race or your background is. They kill you just as dead if you let them – black, white, rich, poor, it doesn't matter. Equal opportunity.

When you begin to realize that everybody's life experience is essentially the same, it gives you a richness of experience you can't get anywhere else.

28
Private detectives and recovery

Or: How to be honest in a sometimes dishonest world

One of the big problems people have after a while in sobriety is the concept of honesty. As the Kipling poem says, "If you can keep your head when all about you are losing theirs and blaming it on you..." Well, in this case, it's how to stay honest when the whole world (it seems) is dishonest and trying to get over on you.

Sometimes people get so fed up that they go back out and use. I've seen it happen. In recovery we call it "poor me, poor me, pour me a drink." Honesty is its own reward. People often forget that. You do the good deed not to get rewarded, but because it's the right thing to do. You don't look for recognition. You remember (some of you) the Lone Ranger. Who was that masked man? Every superhero has a concept of anonymity – Clark Kent, Batman, etc. Why do you think? Because it's part of our collective culture. It goes back to the Bible, in fact; the role of the Good Samaritan.

But what if you do good for people and you get bad in return? Or if you do good and the bad get rewarded? Then what do you do? In short, how do you stay honest and help people in an oftentimes dishonest world?

Well, my friend, it's time for you to meet the existential anti-hero. "The existential *what*?" you say. That's what I said. Now, I'm not an authority on philosophy, but I do know a little bit about it, and I'll share with you what I do know.

Existentialism is a philosophy that became popular after World War II, although its roots go back much farther. Basically, as I understand it, it says you're born, you're going to die, and in between you're responsible for your choices. And since you and you alone are responsible for your choices, you have to be honest with yourself to do the right thing, even if everyone around you is cheating.

The existential anti-hero is someone who has lost his moral center. Joseph Campbell, in his book, *The Hero with a Thousand Faces*, popularized this type of person very well. According to Campbell, the hero is someone who is not in touch with his true feelings and beliefs and through the adventure or journey he realizes what is important in life: the big picture, the grand scheme of things, and changes.

I never intended to get sober. As Clancy, an AA speaker in California, used to say, "I'll play their silly sick game just long enough to get back on my feet, and then adios. But they tricked me," he would go on to say, "and I stayed."

That's what happened to me. I just figured I would go for a while and if it didn't work, I could go back to drinking. Well, I hung around too long, because I got sober instead. You see, through the journey I changed. I realized there was something bigger than myself, a grand scheme of things, and I was only a part – a necessary part, but a part – and that is fine, because now I belong to something meaningful.

I aid in everyone's return from the cliffs of living death, one day at a time. In the movies, you've seen this character a hundred times. In the forties it was Humphrey Bogart in movies like *Casablanca*. "Sure, we love each other, but there is something much bigger than both of us." In modern times it was Harrison Ford's character, Han Solo, in the early *Star Wars* episodes. "Kid, I've been from one end of this galaxy to the next, and if there is a Force, I ain't seen it."

The private detective in the movies fits this role quite well. He sees the corruption but doesn't become engulfed by it, like Jack Nicholson in *Chinatown*. These characters are a bit cynical, a bit jaded, but in the end they win because they know even if the world is corrupt, they are still obligated to do the right thing. This also enables them to see through a lot of the B.S. that goes on in society: the status, money, power, lust, all that stuff that passes off so many times as meaningful.

Well, guess what? You want to be cool and relatively

unintruded much of the time? You want to know how to find your moral center and not be bluffed by a lot of the fluff out there? Well, my friend, work the twelve steps. It ain't perfect but it will give anyone who practices it a true sense of what is truly important in life. Through the journey you may just find out, like me and Clancy, "I'll play their little sick game one more time" – and maybe in the process you will say, "They tricked me," and you too will stay. That's my wish for you.

29
Keep yourself calm for the approaching storm

Calmness is something that doesn't come naturally to me. I came from a family that was high-strung. My father was calm, but my mother was very excitable. As I came into adulthood, I was a sitting duck for addiction. Drinking calmed me down. I'll go so far as to say that all alcoholics are high-strung. At least the ones I've met, and that is one heck of a lot.

So it wasn't until later in my life, when I came across the teachings of the late Dr. Claire Weeks and the twelve steps, along with other things I picked up along the way, like meditation therapy and exercise, that I learned to relax. Today I'm much better at it than I ever was. But I'm still not naturally calm and laid back. People often think when they see me at seminars and book signings that I am naturally, as my young friends would say, "this laid-back dude," but that's not the case. I've had to work hard for all the calm I've got.

One thing that is never talked about among children who

come from alcoholic parents is the difficulty they have in being calm. And yet, calmness is one of the most important traits any human being can have. There is a reason that it is the cornerstone of all the world's major religions. When you're calm you can think clearly. When you're stressed, you're at the mercy of the fight-or-flight response, a very primitive survival mechanism designed to do one of two things: kill or run. It may have served a purpose when we were hunter/gatherers, but it sure gets in the way today with most of what we do.

Also, almost all relapses – be it drugs, alcohol, food, or gambling – occur when people are in a high stress mode. People ask me, do people relapse when they are calm? And my answer to them is no. People are almost always stressed.

In the hundreds and hundreds of people who I have counseled over the years who were relapse-prone, I've never met one who was calm when they relapsed. They were all stressed. They used their addiction to alter their state.

Now, how you calm down is a personal matter. There are many people who have different techniques. Many of them are good. The important point is that you pick one for you, one that works. Trial and error will get you there. When you find something that works for you, keep using it till you get better at it. There is no finer thing you can do for yourself.

To learn to become calm, you must know what it feels like. Only then will you know when you are tense. It took me a long time to understand what calmness felt like. Most of the people I work with are not aware of how tense they are when they first come in to see me. Only after we go through a few stress-reduction exercises are they able to tell.

We live in a world now that seems to get more stressful day by day. Anything you can do to lower your stress without drinking or drugging or going to your addiction of choice will help you in all areas of your life.

30
Stay away from the dark side of recovery

Or: Why, if there is no down, there can be no up

This is a controversial subject. There are those who would have you believe that everything that happens in the rooms of recovery is all peachy-keen. I'm here to tell you that that is not the case. As they say in *Star Wars*, "There is a dark side to the Force." Everybody in recovery came from it. The book *Alcoholics Anonymous* talks about being spiritually sick. When people relapse they go back to the dark side. You can call it relapse, you can call it a spiritual malady, you can call it psychology, you can call it whatever you want. The point is there is an unhealthy side to recovery. You have to have it. It's what makes the whole thing in recovery work. Remember what the meetings are composed of: drunks, drug addicts, people who ran afoul of society's rules.

You have to be careful who you hang around with. We have a saying in recovery: "Hang with the winners." Another way of saying this is hang with those who are sober. Some meetings are better than others. You have to find the ones where you are comfortable and where you feel good about going.

Now, don't get too nervous about what I just said. I know you're thinking, "This guy tells me not to get too nervous, and he's talking about the dark side of the Force. Who is he kidding?" Maybe this will help. There is another saying (I know, all these sayings!): "If you look at twelve-step recovery closely, it's not supposed to work. Too many sick people." But if instead, you identify, don't compare, and look at what you can relate to with people, your fear level will go way down.

In the Orient they talk of the two forces, the Yin and the Yang. In Western religion, we have good and evil. In modern medicine, we talk about health or sickness. I think they're all related. Remember, recovery is mental, physical, and spiritual. So if this little discussion bothers you, then just think about what I'm saying for a minute. And remember that no one really knows how the program of the twelve steps works; only that it does. Think of it like fire. It can cook your food, which is a good thing, but it can burn you, too. No heat, no cold; no good, no bad. You get the picture. Hang with the winners; identify, don't compare; and let the program take care of itself. It will, you know. It's been doing it for a long time.

31

Relapse, stuck points, and how to get out of a rut

As I mentioned before, give an alcoholic a rut and he'll move in and furnish it for you. Getting into a rut is easy; getting out of a rut is tough.

These days, all the talk is about relapse prevention. In relapse prevention training, people are taught to recognize their stuck points. A stuck point is a rut that can get you drunk. Now, everybody has stuck points, but not everybody gets drunk over them.

How you deal with a stuck point will determine whether you stay sober and grow, or relapse and get drunk. Actually, there is a third option, and that is to stay stuck and not drink, at least for a while. And contrary to popular belief, this is where many people that I've observed stay. It's like the old saying, "The devil you know is better than the devil you don't know." So the rut you're in seems okay. Only many times you're not aware that you're depressed. It just seems that's the way it is.

In World War II, when the American Occupation forces rescued the prisoners from the concentration camps, some of the prisoners stayed where they were and refused to come out. The poor fellows had to be coaxed out, because this was what they were familiar with, as bad and horrific as it was.

But staying stuck isn't an option for us either, because if we stay stuck for too long, we will drink or use. So what to do? Well, the answer is simple. (Everything's simple if you know how.) The answer is to go back to basics – home group, sponsor meetings, that sort of thing. Modern research by Stephanie Brown of Stanford University calls them sobriety-based value systems, which is academic talk for "back to basics." Once you re-establish yourself back in your basics, then you can move forward again, but this time you will be much stronger for it. People who are relapse-prone move away from the basics and then use. They forget what got them sober in the first place. Remember, those who forget the past are doomed to repeat it.

Now, what if you're stuck and you don't know it? This is what we call denial. Not all of it is under your conscious control. Not to fear. This is where your support group comes in. As I said earlier, everyone should have someone to talk to about what is bothering them. Guys are at a disadvantage with this, because culturally we are taught not to feel. It's not okay to have any emotion other than anger. So it's important for men and women to have people who confront us in a constructive way when they see we are off course. Examples of this are members of your home group, your sponsor, your friends in recovery, and your counselor. We have another saying in recovery, "If one person says you have a tail, maybe you don't have a tail. But when ten people say you have a tail, then you have a tail."

Relapse is a process, the last stage of which is picking up a drink. I have been in many relapse modes in my time in sobriety, from mild to pretty severe. But what I didn't do (thank God) was pick up a drink or a drug. That's the only mistake that's bad. All the rest can be corrected.

I've had rough times in my sobriety when I walked out the door and couldn't figure out what to do, and then went to a meeting and it passed. And it can pass for you, too, if you think about what we talked about in this section and apply it in your life. Everybody has stuck points in their life. It's just a question of what you do with them when you get them. The choice is yours.

32
Everyone's path is their own

In recovery, like life, everyone has a direction that they take. Some turn left, some turn right, some go straight ahead. Sometimes we make the decision that the person traveling in one direction should change directions to follow us. We think we are going in the right direction. And sometimes we are. If you're sober and the other person is shooting heroin, then it's pretty clear in this particular instance that your direction is correct and his is not. And I know there is a whole school of thought out there today on harm reduction (which, for those of you who don't know, involves getting alcoholics and addicts to use or drink less). But even then, they agree on reducing the quantity and frequency of drug and alcohol consumption.

But in other areas of life, which direction to take is not always that simple. Most of us are confronted with doubt (and oftentimes regrets) over which path we have taken in sobriety or in life. "Maybe I should have married that cute guy/girl some years ago when I had the chance." Or, "Maybe I should have chosen a different career or worked harder on this one." In recovery we call this the coulda-shoulda-woulda syndrome. I coulda done this, I shoulda done that, if only I woulda done that. In short, I regret the path I've taken. If only I could have taken another path in life. And on and on it goes.

This is where the concept comes in that everyone's path is their own. We are all responsible for the paths we take in life. No one else is responsible for them but us. We make the choices as far as the direction we take.

A lot of times people come to me and say, "Barry, you have to set goals," and I don't have any trouble with that. Sure, goals are important. But there is another way of moving through life, and that is by letting go – by opening up to life one day at a time and seeing what unfolds in front of you. I took the most indirect route to becoming a writer you could ever imagine: from active alcoholic, to recovering person, to counselor, to writing programs for courses, to writing my first book to then finding a publisher. I realized I could write when I began to teach. I didn't plan on doing it; it just happened. Sure, I thought about being a writer and I always thought that it would be nice if one day I could write something. But I didn't set off this way or that with a plan. Yes, I know the papers and television are always telling us that this person or that set out at seven with a goal and did it. Some people do that. But most people I have found in sobriety don't know themselves that well. So letting go one day at a time for them is oftentimes the best path.

It doesn't matter so much what path you take, as long as it is meaningful to you. As Don Juan told Carlos Castaneda, "Then ask yourself, and yourself alone, one question ... Does this path have heart? This," he told Carlos, "is the only question you will ever have to ask." I agree.

33

Remember, it's progress, not perfection

Perfectionism is a big killer of sobriety. Believe it or not, more people I've met relapse over not being perfect than almost anything else. "How can this be?" you say. Well, it goes like this. When alcoholics realize that they can't do it perfectly, they decide, "Then I'm not going to do it at all." So for them, it's perfection, not progress. It's the opposite and it doesn't work.

Progress, not perfection, comes from the fifth chapter of the book *Alcoholics Anonymous*, which says, "What an order. I can't go through with it. Remember that we strive for spiritual progress, not spiritual perfection."

What I tell the people I work with is to think of the story of the tortoise and the hare. I ask them to remember who won the race. They think for a minute and then tell me, after giving me a look like, "This is a stupid thing to ask me, this is a child's story." Then they say, "The tortoise won." Right. The tortoise was slow and steady. The hare was fast, but didn't stick to it.

Be a tortoise in sobriety. Lack of patience is a big problem to people in recovery. The opposite of patience (progress, not perfection) is to be demanding, which further translates into "poor me, poor me, pour me a drink" or "I want what I want when I want it – I-I-I me-me-me."

In the book *Twelve Steps and Twelve Traditions*, it says that our happiness in life is in direct proportion to our not making demands on it. Now, a desire is not a demand, as in "a desire to get sober." Or still further in the *Twelve and Twelve*, "The difference between a demand and a request should be obvious to the most casual of observers."

Now, I know what you're thinking. You're saying, "You're the guy who told me not to take no for an answer. Isn't that a contradiction?" I don't think so, although I can see where you might think it is. To quietly with patience not accept no for an answer is the way to go. You can move mountains with that attitude. But it's hard to maintain all the time. I had many periods in my sobriety when only in retrospect I realized I was demanding things. Luckily I had my support networks in place to prevent a major calamity.

So perfectionism can sneak up on any one of us if we are not careful. The important point to remember is that slow is good. That is why in recovery we say, "Easy does it – but do it." Remember, small steady things done over a long period of time will easily beat large efforts done over a short period of time, then dropped.

34
Principles over personalities

This one comes from something called the *twelve principles*. The twelve principles were set up and written by Bill Wilson, the cofounder of AA, and they are the guiding principles of how Alcoholics Anonymous works. I used to think that they only had to do with the organization of the group and had little to do with me living my life outside the rooms. Boy was I wrong.

When you have a group of people as diverse (and oftentimes immature) as alcoholics can be, it's important that we learn to overlook differences that we would never overlook on the outside. Otherwise there would be chaos. One of my old friends in recovery used to say, "It means you check your guns at the door," just like in the old Western movies. Only this is real, and you check your guns of dispute at the door.

In all the years I've been around recovery, in the hallowed halls of meetings, so to speak, nothing has helped me more than this principle. If you can think about it beforehand, it will help to lower your stress, because then when people do things in the meetings that annoy you, it will be easier for you to overlook them. I have seen fights curtailed, grudges ended, and people helped when there was no real love lost between them, all because people in the rooms decided to place principles over personalities.

It can work for you in your personal life, too. Let's say you have a co-worker you can't get along with. Under any other circumstances, you would get in an argument with him or her. But you remember the saying, "principles over personalities" and you remain calm. Another argument is avoided. You realize that the common principle is working together as a team. If you're married, the common principle is the marriage. If it's your family, the common principle is your family.

Early on, I used to go to a lot of meetings that were pretty gruff. Some of them looked like motorcycle rallies for an outlaw biker gang. But with all that testosterone flying, there were rarely if ever any confrontations. "Why is that?" you ask.

Well, I know why. Because of principles over personalities, that's why. Group unity was the most important thing. And because of this, people in the rooms overlooked their individual differences. And believe me, if these groups could get along, anyone can get along.

When you decide to put this concept into your life, a lot of your problems drop by the wayside. And if you get stressed, you will know what to do to get back on course. You were probably personalizing something that didn't need to be personalized. And when things become less personal to you, you and I, and all of us become happier, healthier, calmer people.

35

No pain, no gain

If there is one group of people who will do almost anything to avoid pain, it is addicts and alcoholics. We will do almost anything not to have to deal with reality. But in so doing, we create more pain for ourselves. By doing drugs or drinking or overeating or gambling, our problems magnify. Also, we become weak, because rather than deal with our problems, we learn to drink or use.

On the other hand, when you go through a problem and you don't drink or use, you become stronger. Your nervous system is in many ways like a muscle. And like a muscle, when you lift weights, over time if there is enough rest between workouts, your muscles get stronger. So it is with your nerves. When you stress, when drug free, then you rest, and then stress them again, you get stronger. You go to the meeting, you're nervous, you come home, rest, watch TV, whatever. The next night you go again, you're slightly less nervous. Eventually, over time, if you don't drink, you get more confident, calmer, more in control. But you had to go through the pain to get there. No pain, no gain.

We now live in a world where instant calm is the order of the day. No one wants to work for anything anymore. That's the danger of drugs and alcohol. Through them, we can achieve instant calm. But one of the main problems – not the only problem – is that drugs and alcohol (and for many, food) cover up the pain. It's like seeing the light come on in the dashboard of your car and you put tape over it. You think because the tape covers up the red light, that you don't have any trouble with the car anymore. You and I know this is not true, but that is what people think when they partake of their particular addiction.

When you live your life on life's terms, you actually, over time, have less pain because you're not avoiding the necessary pain of life. Not to get too egg-headed here, but even Sigmund Freud in his writing said that neurosis is the avoidance of *necessary* suffering.

When people come into treatment where I work, they have legal, medical, and emotional problems. Many of them are homeless and unemployed. They don't want to face their pain. You know what I tell them? "Pick the biggest problem first and work on it. Then pick the second biggest and work on that, and so on until you've faced all your problems." You know what they almost always tell me? They are surprised at how much better they feel and how they are in less pain.

Pain – emotional distress – is the entryway into a new life. There is a saying in recovery that's not said much anymore, "Recovery doesn't open up the gates of heaven and let you in; it opens up the gates of hell to let you out." Face your pain and get out of hell.

One thing I've learned in recovery is that you can do anything sober that you could do drunk. That means you can face all your fears sober and they won't overwhelm you. You can trust me on this one. I've had all kinds of problems in sobriety, some big, some small, some in-between. But one thing, thank God, I learned. You don't have to drink or take your particular addiction to get through life.

As the saying goes, "What doesn't kill you makes you stronger." When you go through your particular pain and don't pick up, as we say in sobriety, "You will know a new peace and a new happiness." All pain passes if you don't pick up. If you're digging, don't stop until you hit the treasure. One shovelful of dirt after you feel like quitting could be the one where your shovel hits the treasure box and you hear that *clunk, clunk.* The treasure is your freedom. No finer treasure could ever be in your possession. Pain is your entryway. Claim the treasure. It is yours.

36

Crooks, con artists, cheats and hustlers:

Some of my best teachers, and how they can be your teachers, too (for the good)

When my life stretches out in front of me and I look back on the things I have learned and the people who have taught me the most, I have to say, right up there with all the rest, I have to put con artists as some of my best teachers. Now what I mean by con artists, for the most part, is reformed con artists, generally people in recovery. So actually, to be more precise, you could call them ex-con artists. The point is that most of them were far from the fields of academia or established professions.

Why did I find these people so effective as teachers? Number one, is that many of them were dynamic presenters. They could say things or write things (usually say) that could put light on a situation or problem that had been previously troubling to me. All the pieces would seem to fit after they got through explaining it.

Here are a couple of examples: Bob E., who I mentioned earlier, used to say, "The madness only makes sense as long as I keep it between my ears. As soon as I tell someone what I'm thinking, I can see how crazy it is." I never got why it was so important to share until I heard him say it.

Liz B., another prominent AA speaker from the East Coast, used to say "from Park Avenue to the park bench" when she was describing who could be affected by alcoholism. No one was immune.

Now here's my point. Bob E. was a convicted felon and Liz B. had her own story of misery and then recovery that was every bit as extraordinary as Bob's. I had been to all kinds of therapists, counselors, and doctors before I came in contact with people like this.

I've argued this point with academics for years. Some people have a talent for reaching you, talking to you, entering your world. Bob E. and people like him, early on in my recovery and still to a large extent today, had the capacity of motivating me to do things that *nobody else* – and I mean nobody– could get me to do.

And they weren't all famous people either. Many of them were just average local people like you and me. Now, I don't want to get into the debate of whether or not alcoholics are chosen people are not, but I will say this: (We are certainly fortunate) if you hear some people tell you this early on in your sobriety (as I did) and you take it as a force to do good (as I did), it can do the most amazing things for you. It can pick you up off the garbage heap of humanity and place you right where you have to be, to be happy and successful.

You can call it a cult, you can call it brainwashing, you can call it whatever you want. When a person can talk to you and enter your world and motivate you, they can help you do the most amazing things. When there is no hope, hope is given. Then if you hang in there long enough, that magical feeling will come over you that says, "If he can do it, I can do it." And if you get that, you're on your way, because then you will know, like me, that another con artist has succeeded and touched you. Thank God!

37

You've got to go to any length

Or: Why half-measures don't work

In every Alcoholics Anonymous meeting across the county, they read something from the fifth chapter of the book *Alcoholics Anonymous*. It goes like this: "If you have decided you want what we have and are willing to go to any length to get it, then you're ready to take certain steps." And later it says, "Half measures availed us nothing." Two good sayings: "willing to go to any length" and "half measures availed us nothing."

These two phrases changed the course of my life and the lives of thousands of people who have listened to them and acted on them over the years. It can change the course for you if you let it.

Early on in my recovery I grasped the meaning of being willing to go to any length. It was after my first relapse. I experienced what alcoholics call a moment of clarity. The thought was, "You weren't working the program, you only thought you were." I realized "weren't working the program" and "half measures" were the same thing. That changed my life.

I was coming off of almost ten years of drinking and drugs, the worst of which were prescription drugs. There was no way I was going to make it without going to any length. I had one of the best doctors helping me – Dr. Claire Weeks, the famous Australian physician – and I still had trouble. Without "going to any length," forget it.

People often ask me what constitutes "any length" and the answer I give them is simple. It means anything that is not illegal, immoral, or unethical. Robbing a bank is clearly out, as is lying to your best friend. But everything else counts. We often hear a saying, "Your addiction doesn't care what excuse you give it. If it wants you to get a craving, you get a craving."

So, you might have to go to ninety meetings in ninety days; you might have to go to two meetings a day for a while if you're not working. You might have to call nine people before you get that tenth person on the phone. I'll tell you one thing I know: You will have to push yourself longer and harder than anything you will know up to that point, and then push it through out the other side. But when you hit the other side, you will know you have made it. On that particular problem, you would have bought yourself another little piece of freedom. More freedom, more life. Well, you get the picture.

38
The Rip van Winkle effect and what it has to do with sobriety

When I sobered up, I felt like Rip van Winkle. You know, the guy from the Washington Irving story who fell asleep and awoke twenty years later with a long gray beard. I didn't have the long gray beard, but I could identify with him. Things felt out of sync. There was a whole decade that I couldn't account for. And that line in the third step from the book *Twelve Steps and Twelve Traditions* which states, "Panic takes over our friend when he thinks of all the bridges to safety alcohol burned behind him" – that was me. I felt out of it, lost, like some alien from a distant planet placed here on Earth, far away from home. It took years for me to get comfortable with being back on Earth. I had been gone a long time, just like Rip van Winkle.

We often speak of this in recovery. We call non-recovering people Earth people, people of the place we're coming back to.

Even today there are times when I feel like I don't fit in. But it's less than it used to be and it always passes if I let it.

The point is, we are all Rip van Winkles, all lost to our own addictions. We have all (most of us) been asleep for quite a while. Then, as if through some magical intervention, we have come alive all at once to walk the face of the Earth again. The prayers that you had, that I had, that said, "Please give me one more chance," have been answered, and you were spared one more time to walk the land of the living – to have sunlight on your face and hope in your heart and meaning in your life. How you prayed for this chance, and now it has come. Although you feel grateful, you also feel strange. Everybody left a long time ago – careers, marriage, death, the whole drama of life. And you and I were asleep.

What of those bridges to safety that alcohol burned behind us? They are gone. Echoes in our mind. So you let go of your fantasies of what might have been and get on with what you have. You get out of your own way. Let go, "Let God," as we say. You don't even know if you believe in God, but you do it anyway, just to feel better. A little at first, then for longer durations, one step at a time. And then one day, for a small part of the day, maybe only a few minutes, you feel better. You don't understand it, but you feel the relief. You let go again and you feel better again, and so it goes. You've let go and nothing bad has happened to you.

The Rip van Winkle effect, for the time being, has been put to rest. You no longer feel like an alien in a strange land. You experience some peace of mind. Maybe not for long, but a little bit. Coming back from the dead is never easy (the walking dead of our addictions) and leaving the ghosts of the past is never easy either. But it can be done, one day at a time, if you let it and get out of your way, letting God – the universe, nature, the program, whatever you believe in – take effect. Until one day, when you're sitting at work or home or out and you get this feeling that wasn't there before. It's not just on the surface, but goes all the way through you. And you realize (surprise, surprise) that "Hey, I really belong. This is my place, my planet, my people, and I am a part of them and I deserve to be here." And you realize, maybe for the first time in your life, that it's good to be back. No longer an alien in a strange land. You belong. It's a great feeling to have. Welcome home.

39

How to live a long life in sobriety

Or: Why, when most people sober up, it takes a bullet to kill them

"Living a long life in sobriety, what is he talking about with this one?" you say. Well, let me tell you this: For many people who sober up the right way (and that's a big if – the right way), for those people, as my old mentor Jess Lair used to say, it takes a bullet to kill them.

They get healthy, even if they smoke, which I don't advocate (they usually quit when they are sober a while). When people get sober, things tend to fall in place for them one step at a time. "What does sobriety have to do with aging?" you may ask. Good question. It is this: One of the strongest indications of aging has been mental health, which is sobriety. In George Valliant, MD's classic study on aging, he found that for all other variables holding constant (other things that affect aging), the strongest indicator of who would live the longest was a person's mental health.

Sobriety is mental health with a spiritual component. So getting sober, working the twelve steps to the best of your ability, will also help you live a long life. By the way, this finding – that mental health is the strongest predictor of longevity – has now held constant for twenty years and has resisted all attempts by researchers to refute it.

The ancient mystics believed that most people would grow old and die because they watched other people grow old and die. In recovery, if one is working their program, there is a large part of them that stays young spiritually and mentally. And as we have already said, staying young mentally helps you stay young physically.

Many people, as they get older, get bitter. They have resentments, and resentments turn into bitterness, and bitterness turns into regrets, and from regrets it's a short hop, step, and a jump to depression.

Hell, I know young people who are bitter, so it doesn't necessarily have to do with age, except many of us unfortunately wind up like Bigger Thomas in Richard Wright's novel, *Native Son*, where he says, "The will to live has been beaten out of me." That is what addiction is. It beats the will to live out of us. That's if we let it. It doesn't have to be. 'Cause once, you should have died but didn't. As Dustin Hoffman's character says in *Little Big Man*, "You ain't never the same again." That's what it means to have a spiritual awakening. You ain't never the same again.

I've never been the same after I sobered up. I never took life for granted anymore. It was all precious to me. Why? Because it was almost taken from me. And it was almost taken from you. Most likely, if you're reading this book, you're on your own spiritual journey.

So how do you retain this youth, this mental health, this sacredness? Well, I hate to harp on an old theme, but one way several million people have done it is to work the twelve steps. Yes, there are other techniques. As I've said before, many people have used this technique and as they say, "If it ain't broke, don't fix it."

I have seen many people who have been sick and have died while going to meetings – died of cancer and other things. But I have also seen other sick people who, after a period of time, got well, and for some of them their cancer went into remission. Now, I'm not saying that the twelve steps are a cure for cancer. I'm not saying that cancer isn't a devastating illness. My mother died of cancer, and I often thought if she had some type of twelve-step program, it might have helped her to live a longer life. And some of you might say that I'm using statistical preference to just choose the examples that I want, and that is a fair comment, too. All I'm trying to do is share with you what I have seen with my own eyes.

Let me tell you a story. There was this English chap I knew in recovery. His name was Arty. I knew Arty for years in recovery, and then I lost track of him. One day I saw Arty again. He looked terrible. I said, "What's wrong?" Arty said, "I have cancer. They gave me three months to live."

What do you say to that? Nothing. I just listened and told him I would pray for him. After that, I lost track of Arty. Then one day a few years later, I ran into Arty again. He looked different, but I didn't know why. Finally I said, "Arty, you look different. How are you feeling?" He said, "Great, I don't have cancer anymore."

"Really?" I was surprised; the last time I saw him, he looked half-dead.

"When the doctor told me that I had only a few months to live, I said, what the heck. I might as well go to meetings. So that's what I did. I went to a meeting every day, and figured I would get right with my higher power. When I went back for a check-up a few months later, the doctor was surprised. The cancer had receded a bit. The doctor didn't know what to think. Eventually the cancer went into remission. Now it's been over two years and the doctor told me that if I make it a bit longer, that it will be formally in remission." Arty and I both looked at each other. We knew what had happened. Arty had surrendered to his problem and by surrendering, giving up, to God's will (reality), he went into remission.

You think this is crazy talk? William Glasser, MD, in his book *Control Theory*, states that we all have an internal robot in us that controls our inner functions, and when we get out of control, our body responds to things like cancer. Glasser advocated activities that give the person a sense of control;

meditation and running were two examples he gave. How about twelve-step meetings?

We – you and I – have far more control over ourselves than we know. Use the program to help you live a long, healthy life and you too will know what it means when they say it takes a bullet to kill him.

40
Be serious but don't get too serious

When people stop alcohol, drugs, or other addictions, they start to take their life seriously – oftentimes too seriously. Why is this? Well, I think there are a couple of reasons. One is that when people say they have contacted a higher power of their own understanding, what happens to many of them is that the God of their understanding often becomes the God of their childhood. The God of understanding and compassion becomes the God of fire and brimstone.

Most of this is unconscious, however, so people are not really aware of what they are truly thinking. Words like fun and sex and laughter often get put on the back burner. And although many people formally take the view that addiction is a disease, that we are sick people getting well, not bad people getting good, they often subconsciously take the view that they are bad people trying to get good. They put a moral view on it. And instead of taking healthy chances with calculated risks to help them enjoy life more, these people use words like "I have to work on myself more," "I'm not ready for that," "That's not me," "I'm a spiritual person." All this, while the world passes them by. They get too serious.

Life is a serious process. It's good to be serious. But it's not good to be too serious. Neurosis is essentially taking ourselves and others too seriously. There is an absence of humor. As I said, these types of people don't laugh much. They read endless self-help books and overly focus on early childhood problems that may or may not have a bearing on what is currently happening. If you had to ask me one of the downsides of long-term twelve-step involvement, I would have to say that for many of us, it's taking ourselves too seriously.

So what is the antidote? For one, it's getting some humor back in our lives. Laughter is an important component of sobriety and life. If there is humor and laughter, then the overly critical thinking faculty, which we all have, is temporarily suspended. We see the light side of things and we have fun.

The other thing many of us have to do is to look at what our higher power means to us. Is it really as I understand him, her, or it? Or is it influenced by things I learned from childhood? For many of us, this has to do with sex. Sex is pleasure and many of us in recovery are conflicted about what constitutes legitimate pleasure. Guilt comes in two forms: earned and unearned. Earned guilt comes when we do something wrong, and unearned guilt comes when we feel guilty over something that is not our fault.

If we don't learn how to laugh, we are in trouble. Laughter

is a part of life. Learn to see the sunlight. So that in the end you and I can remember what it really means to not take ourselves too seriously.

41

Thou shalt make thyself comfortable at the lower level before moving to the next higher level

Whenever I want to move to a new higher level of accomplishment or development, I first try to make myself comfortable at the lower level that I know. Earlier I said you don't always have to be comfortable, but bear with me on this one.

Although this concept is similar to the earlier discussion of how to avoid stuck points, it's not quite the same thing.

Making yourself comfortable at a lower level is a way of life. Dealing with stuck points has more to do with relapse prevention. What's the difference, you say? It seems contradictory, but as I've said, sometimes life is contradictory. Sometimes you do one thing and sometimes you do something else. Being comfortable on the lower level involves more of a broad-brush approach. It involves making yourself comfortable over the long haul, not just over a specific event.

I've had many periods in my life where I tried to push through to some higher level – work, career, social – and I wound up falling flat on my face because I didn't try to secure the lower level. Maybe it was not going to enough meetings. Maybe I wasn't talking to my friends enough. Maybe it was something else. In any event, I found over time (usually a short amount of time) I wound up crazier than a bedbug. Sometimes I found myself sitting in my kitchen, drinking my morning coffee, realizing that I felt like chewing on a table leg. All because I pushed too fast and didn't take care of what we call in the program, "first things first."

As it says in the book *Twelve Steps and Twelve Traditions*, "The difference between a demand and a simple request is plain to anyone." Oftentimes we have a strong desire to move up and to better ourselves. And oftentimes we attempt to move up without stabilizing the last camp below. When you climb mountains, so I'm told, you have to secure the lower-level camp before you move on to the summit. So it is with life: one step at a time, one thing at a time. Don't go too fast, just keep going. Just make sure you're relatively comfortable where you're at. That's why friends are so important. When you network with your friends, you can share your feelings with each other, your frustrations, as well as your hopes.

If you work on it, you can get to a feeling that says, "Enough, I feel satisfied. I am comfortable," the way you oftentimes feel after a very good meal. Only now it's with friends, and when you get this way and feel it, you will be ready for the next higher level because you have now secured the lower level. Only now you won't be desperate and you will, therefore, be much more likely to get what you want.

42
Remember your primary purpose

In the book *Twelve Steps and Twelve Traditions*, one of the traditions states that, "our primary purpose is to stay sober and help other alcoholics to achieve sobriety." This is an interesting phrase, "primary purpose." Notice they don't say *only* purpose. Primary purpose, as in the most important one. You have other purposes – job, family, social – but you place primary purpose on your recovery. So it would look something like this: recovery one, job two; or recovery one, family two, job three. At any rate, you get the idea.

"Well, what about putting family behind recovery?" you say. Look at it this way: If you have ever flown in a commercial airplane and you have heard the instructions on how to use the oxygen mask in case of an emergency, you will notice that the flight attendant tells you to place the mask on yourself first before you put it on your child, if you have a child with you. Why is that? Because if you pass out, you won't be able to put the oxygen mask on anybody. So the message is you first. First you save your life, then you save other people's lives. So it is here in recovery. Primary purpose: First your recovery, then the other things. Your recovery is your oxygen, your lifeblood. With it you have everything, and without it you have nothing. So primary purpose is important.

Another way to think of primary purpose is devotion to your own personal growth. That's what they mean when they say you come first. Your growth comes first, one day at a time.

Some things are simple. When people I've counseled relapse, it's at least partly because they didn't pay attention to this saying. When you think of primary, think of prioritize: to come first or to make it your goal.

Remember, primary doesn't mean only or obsessive. It simply means the most important thing for you. I've had many a time in my life when I was in some difficult situation and I didn't know what to do, and I remembered my primary purpose: not my job, not my family, but my sobriety. I had to put the oxygen mask on me first if I was to help anyone else.

There is a little bell that goes off in my head when I'm in enough pain, and it says move on, do something. And a little bell should go off in your head too for you to do something – remember your primary purpose and take action. I know you can do it.

43
Thou shalt have a life outside of recovery

I have a saying, "The second biggest problem people have is not going to enough meetings; and the biggest problem people have is going to too many." Now, I'm not talking to people who are retired or who go to a lot of meetings because they want to. I'm talking about a whole other group of people I see who go to too many meetings for the wrong reasons. We have a saying in recovery, "Don't drink and go to meetings (or don't use drugs and go to meetings or don't eat compulsively and go to meetings)." Now, this is fine in the beginning, but after a while we have to do something different. We have already discussed the concept of Earth people. Earth people, remember, are people who are not in recovery.

For years I used to say Earth people didn't understand me – and some of them may not have – but recovering people did. There is nothing really wrong with this on the surface. And for a time in sobriety, I think it is necessary to surround oneself with just recovering people. God knows I did it for years. The only problem is that you miss out on a lot that life has to offer. You can even lose your competitive edge in life, thinking that everyone is like all the people you know in recovery. It's a big world out there, and meetings are a bridge back to life, not a halfway point in between.

A study was done a few years ago on the one trait people shared who had successfully survived catastrophic situations – divorce, bankruptcy, major illness, death of a spouse, etc. The investigators thought they would find IQ, education, things like that. But what they found was people who survived catastrophic setbacks and did the best were people who had multiple interests. When one interest fell off, they picked up another one. They worked out; they went to meetings; they talked to their friends; they had their careers or jobs. You get the picture.

So what are your interests? Oh, you don't have any? Well, it's time to get some. What do you like to do? What did you do in the past that you don't do anymore? What have you never done that you would like to try? Maybe it's something that you are already doing that you would like to continue doing. Whatever it is, take a piece of paper and write it down. Pick two of the things out and start to work on them. Maybe you want to take up scuba diving, maybe play golf. Maybe you want to go back to school. Whatever it is, pursue it. I've been working out almost as long as I've been sober, and I can't tell you how much this has helped me over the years. It's given me something else to do. And it's given me a body in the process –

"lean and mean," as they say. Now that's my thing. You find out what is good for you, then do it. Find out what else works and do that.

What you will find in time is that you will have your own separate recovery program through the hobbies that you do. This will give you a renewed source of strength and confidence. So that one day down the road, you will realize that life is recovery and recovery is life. And that Earth people are not separate from us. They are us and we are them – all one.

44
When you're green, you grow; when you're ripe, you rot

They often used to say in recovery, "When you're green, you grow; when you're ripe, you rot." What exactly does this mean? Well, look at it this way. You're either moving toward sobriety and growth or you're going backward toward where you came from, toward your addiction – and for many of us, death. "Green" refers to keeping your memory green. The old-timers when I was coming up used to say, "The weller I am, the sicker I was." What that means is the longer I'm sober, the more I can remember about my past. This is good as long as we don't use it as an excuse to beat ourselves up.

When you remember where you came from, you remember where you want to go. And when you get in a bad space, you remember that you have to change. You have to grow and, for most of us, to keep growing. "Grow or die," as we used to say when I came around. If you don't want to sweep the floor after the meeting, do it, because if you don't, you will die. That's how I was taught. It may seem harsh to some of you, but there is a cold, hard reality to it. When we are ever mindful of where we came from, we grow; and when we become complacent, we die.

And the worst type of death is the walking dead. Most of us have been dead on our feet in our addiction, and a few of us in sobriety. I don't have to say any more about it. It's a bad place to be. Growth is better.

So pain comes in two forms: the pain of death (rotting) and the pain of growth. Growth requires pain, but it's good pain because it leads to the resolution of conflict or a problem. But when we are in our addictions, the pain is colored with hopelessness and despair, and that is the worst. There is no sunlight down there, only darkness.

So keep on the path of your own recovery. Look at the light coming and know that it is daylight and not a train coming the other way. As Morgan Freeman's character says in the movie *The Shawshank Redemption*, "Either get busy living or get busy dying."

I was dead on my feet for a long time and I never want to go back there. That's what they mean when they say, "My worst day sober is better than my best day drunk." Because even in the worst of it in sobriety, there is hope. In the active addiction, we knew we were killing ourselves slowly for some of us and fast for a few.

At meetings, if the meetings are run right, we say what it was like, what happened, and what it's like now. We talk about how we used to rot – how we almost rotted out, hit bottom, and then how we started to grow. This sequence, taken and applied, is a very powerful technique for change, for growth, and for life. My wish for you is that you use it and may you always choose life.

45
If you want to learn something, teach it to someone else

One of the best ways to learn something is to teach it to someone else. This is one of the benefits of volunteer work in general and twelve-step work in particular. We have all heard the story of the Good Samaritan from the Bible. In modern times, it would be the equivalent of someone being mugged and then some stranger coming along and getting the person medical attention, and then getting the person a room to stay in until his wounds healed. That, as many of you know, is where we get the term "Good Samaritan" from. In twelve-step programs, this is the twelfth step: to help another addict.

There is a good feeling that comes from helping people. We have a saying in recovery, "If I have a problem and I help you with your problem, then I have half a problem." The secondary benefit of helping someone is that I learn on a deeper level that which I'm teaching.

If the person has trouble not drinking or not partaking of the particular substance to which he or she is addicted, if you help that particular person stay sober, you have just helped yourself stay sober longer. As another recovery saying goes, "I've sponsored a lot of people. Not all of them are sober, but I'm sober."

Therefore, we really help someone not so much for them but for us. It's selfish – selfish in a good way. We help them because it helps us. In recovery, we practice being the Good Samaritan in our daily lives; if not with everybody we meet, at least with those people we meet in recovery.

I remember early on in my recovery, crazy as hell, I would help everybody. Why, I would help you even if you didn't want to be helped. But you know what? It helped me, and I began the long, difficult climb back to the world of the living. The other world was the world of the living dead. Helping someone move from the world of the living dead to the world of the living ensures that you stay alive and sober one more day. You see, the living dead aren't zombies in the movies. They walk among us every day in the form of addiction: Hell. Free the person from their addiction and you help bring one more person back to life. There is no finer calling you could have.

People often ask me what I do for a living. I tell them I'm a garbage picker. They look at me strangely when I tell them this. I then tell them that I pick people up off the garbage heap of humanity, show them the elusive quality of their own self-worth, inform them that (often unbeknownst to them) they were taking some poison that was keeping them enslaved, and then I help move them on their way again.

So what's the moral of this story? If you feel like using, find someone else to help. Teach someone else what you have learned about recovery. Don't do it for any rewards; just do it for you. So that you will stay sober one more day.

Secondarily, do you have trouble with depression, anxiety, anger, shame, you name it? Help someone out with his or her problems and I guarantee you will see an improvement in this area in yourself.

Maybe instead of inner things, you have trouble with outer things. You have a problem going to meetings? Take someone to a meeting with you. You have trouble sharing at meetings? Encourage someone else to share. As a side benefit, you will start to share more yourself.

The way out of darkness toward the light is never easy for any of us. Help someone see the true brightness of recovery by teaching them something they need to know to save their life and you will be rewarded in ways that you could never imagine. You will know the true meaning of the story of the Good Samaritan.

46

Make a friend of fear, or at least don't make it your enemy

Fear is our constant companion. It is either full-bore in front of us in a crisis or lingering out there off in the distance. A lot of us in our modern life forget this. We've become sanitized with home entertainment systems, air conditioning, and shopping malls, to name a few. We think we are sheltered from ever having to be afraid. But as the old saying goes, "Everybody is afraid of something." In addition to alcoholism, which is just fear in disguise, fear takes many shapes, sizes, and forms. It can be overeating, gambling, excessive accumulation of wealth, drug addiction, antisocial acting out and phobias, depression – the list goes on and on. There is a reason that fear is bracketed as the main character defect in the book *Alcoholics Anonymous*.

The opposite of fear is courage. Winston Churchill said that courage is the master virtue, making all other virtues possible.

Eddie Rickenbacker, the famed World War I flying ace, said courage was doing the thing you were afraid to do while you were afraid. He said that if you weren't afraid, then you couldn't feel courage. A lot of people confuse fearlessness with courage. They're not the same thing. We all feel fear. It's what we do with it that counts.

If you had to ask me the person who taught me the most about fear, it wasn't a guy or a military hero. It was a woman. A grandmotherly woman, to be exact. When I first came in contact with this person, she was in her seventies. Her name was Dr. Claire Weekes, and she was from Australia. What she taught me about fear changed my life. Fear can be either real or imagined. Either way, it's an extremely uncomfortable feeling to deal with. What did I learn about courage from this little old woman? She taught me that if you want something bad enough, you would have the courage.

Think about something that you want more than anything else you could imagine. Feel it there in the pit of your stomach. There: That's where courage is – in your stomach, not in your head. It's a good place for it. It gives strength to your backbone, she would say. No one had ever explained it to me this way before.

We all have fear. We all have something we are afraid of. You may not have the all-encompassing fear I had of prescription drug dependence and drinking, but we all have things we are afraid of. To be human is to be afraid. And there is no shame in it. It's not whether or not you're afraid; it's what you do with it that counts.

When I first did the exercise above, the only thing I could think of that I wanted was to get well. *That* I could feel in my gut.

What do you feel in your gut? What keeps you stuck? What do you want to accomplish that you don't think you could ever accomplish? What do you desire? Look deep into that desire; that's where you will find your courage. Feel that feeling in your stomach. That is where it is. That feeling will enable you to accomplish whatever you need to do. Feel it, claim it. It's yours, a gift from the Creator, if you will. Make it your friend when you face your fear so that fear itself doesn't have to be the enemy.

47
Don't be bluffed by the odds; remember you are unique

These days everything is the odds. Odds for this, odds for that. The odds on how many people will make it into recovery. How many people will relapse. How many people will stay in the program. How many people will drop out.

When you think of all this, rather than get hypnotized by it and get discouraged, remember that you are a work in progress. You are becoming a different person every day if you are working on yourself. And although you don't want to be overly optimistic, you don't want to be overly negative either. You focus on *you* and what you can do, and let the odds take care of themselves.

That's what I had to do. The odds were not in my favor. I had been sick for too long. Most people who are down as far as I was don't come back. I know that now. But here's the point: I'm not the odds, and neither are you. Each person is unique.

The philosopher and novelist Ayn Rand did not think very much of the odds. She used to say that rather than focus on what people could be and ought to be, we focus on the odds – and all they do is tell what an average group of people can accomplish. In short, we have made odds the end-all and be-all in life, rather than focusing on someone's potential. In twelve-step parlance, this results in making odds your higher power.

Arthur DeVany, professor emeritus in economics at the University of California at Irvine, calls occurrences that we talk about extraordinary events. This would include things like the Beatles, Harry Potter, *Titanic* (the movie) – things that occur that become so popular that no one would or could have predicted. They have occurred throughout history, going back as far or farther than the rise of Christianity, a small (at the time) religion that, as we all know, spread throughout the world.

Recovery, for some people, is an extraordinary event. No one could have predicted where some people would wind up on the road to sobriety. So you shouldn't ignore the odds, and you shouldn't be hypnotized by them either.

What is the extraordinary event in your life? What are you capable of doing that you didn't think you could do? Remember, if one person has done it, then you probably can do it, too. That is the basis of twelve-step treatment. You hear one person's recovery, and you then conclude that if he recovered, then I (you) can recover, too. That's how I did it. And that's how many, many other people have done it. It's called the power of example. But it's not some infomercial on television.

What you're seeing when you go to a meeting is a real live person.

In substance abuse treatment, many people are told only three out of thirty will get sober. You know what I tell them? You all can get sober. I ask them, how many people are allowed as children to go to school? They tell me all children, because education is mandatory in America. Then I ask them, "How many children are allowed to graduate grammar school without being able to read."

They say, "None."

I say, "Why?"

They say, "Because everybody who is in sound health can be taught to read."

I say to them, "The technology exists to teach people to read. How many of you would allow it, if you were told by the school that your child was going to graduate illiterate? You would never put up with it. So, why would you put up with your own relapse? Just like there is zero tolerance for illiteracy in America, you need zero tolerance for your own failure, your own relapse – because the technology exists for your own recovery."

Screw the odds. Instead focus on what you know you can do, and let the odds take care of themselves. The results will surprise you.

48

The joy is in the journey

Or: Why it's longer and harder than the self-help books tell you it is

When I first came into recovery, they used to tell me that the joy was in the journey, not the destination. They don't say this much anymore in the rooms, where everything is focused on success and goals and having things.

Don't let the Zen-like simplicity of this saying fool you. This is one of those concepts whose power comes from its simplicity. "Why is this?" you say. Because through the journey, the adventure, the recovery process – you change. What you do on your path to where you want to go is almost as important – or more important – than the goal you achieve.

"Are you saying that goals aren't important?"

No, goals are important. Just don't fall in love with them. The journey is equally important. You see, when we are in our addiction, we don't look at things this way. We have no patience. Everything is "I want this now." And if I don't get it, it's terrible. But in recovery, we learn that through the process of the struggle we change and grow. And you can have a good time doing it. Some of my fondest memories in life were when I was in early recovery, when I had nothing. It didn't matter. I experienced the joy of being let out of hell, sitting in diners after meetings, talking to other people in recovery. I have no finer memories.

There is another reason for focusing on the journey. This is because the journey will probably be longer and harder than you thought. If you can focus on the journey, then things get much easier. Part of the title of this essay is, "It's longer and harder than the self-help books told you," and I should add, "But you can do it." Most self-help books suffer from one thing, and that is they are overly optimistic. Remember, having too much confidence is just as bad as having not enough. In recovery, overconfidence can kill you. That is why people in the recovery community have always cautioned people away from the traditional self-help fare.

But let me tell you what can happen when you take a realistic view of life and of recovery. You settle down, you focus on the journey, you pay attention to the task at hand, and then you move out across the terrain of your existence one step at a time. And as the old saying goes, "A journey of a thousand miles must begin with a single step."

You're marching, you're marching, and focusing on where you put your next step, and then, as if the Higher Power has answered, he or she gives you what you want: the relationship, the job, the promotion. It comes to you. And it usually comes from the least expected sources. You will look over there to your right and it will come from the left. You look left and it will come from the right. You look up and it will come from below.

Just stay on the path, and if you get diverted and get off the path, that's okay. As soon as you realize it, get back on course and start walking. One day you will look back and realize you have changed. You have become stronger – forged in steel, if you will – able to do things you never thought you could do before: handle stress, confront your fears, solve problems, you name it.

There is nothing like a little adversity in a person's life to make a stronger, better person. And one day, you will look out over the landscape of your life and instead of seeing a burned-out, barren wasteland, you will see one that is lush and green, and the sun will be shining. And you will smile to yourself because, you realize, that is the light of recovery. And this time you realize it is shining on you.

49
Don't blame; focus on solutions

"Addicts blame; winners focus on solutions," or so it is said in recovery circles. But how many of us really do that?

Just before people relapse, they get into a blaming mood. Everything is wrong, nothing is right. In this state, we tend to see ourselves as victims, unable to change, stuck. A victim of circumstances that are beyond our control to change. Or so we think. But is this the way it really is?

All change starts with us. As soon as we start to change one thing, we can break the pattern in the blame cycle. The changes can be small. But what is important to know is that when we change anything, we start to change ourselves. We move from the blame game to being solution oriented.

"What about true injustice?" you say. "Aren't you supposed to be mad at that? Childhood problems, societal indiscretions – are you saying we shouldn't get mad?"

No, that's not what I'm saying. Sure, you can get mad. But sooner or later, we have to come out of it, and when we do, we have to look for a way out – to focus on the path we are going to take through the destruction.

I had an old therapist who, every time I would get on one of my "he did this" and "she did that" and "society did this" routines, he would say, "But that's not helping you. You have to focus on solutions."

When he said that, a little bell would go off in my head and I would think, "He's not telling me I don't have a problem. He's just telling me that blaming won't help me." It would be like the rewind button on a tape recorder was pushed and my mind would stop. Then I could press play, and I could focus on solutions.

"Where does venting my anger come in?" you say. "Don't I have to get it off my chest?"

Yes and no.

Certainly venting has its place. But it's overrated. In the recovery community, during the last twenty years, venting one's emotions has been granted to a very high status. The truth is, sometimes you have to vent and sometimes you don't. But what you do have to do, almost always, is focus on solutions. Too many of us these days, it seems to me, vent and blame and leave it at that, under the mistaken belief that this will help. It won't.

In twelve-step meetings, there is a pattern that we use to express our problems. It goes like this: How it was, what happened, and what it's like now. How it was – I drank. My life was bad. What happened – I wound up in a detox. What it's like now – I'm in recovery and my life is good, and it's now manageable.

Too many meetings these days go like this: How it was, what happened – and that's it. No "what it's like now." What it's like now is the solution part of your recovery. I call the types of meetings where they stay on "what happened" only "group depression meetings," where you feel worse after you leave the meeting than you did before you started.

This is not for you. What you want is, "what I'm going to do differently." As we say in recovery, "Insanity is doing the same thing over and over again, expecting different results." Do the thing differently. Change one thing. Focus on the situation, then how you can change it, and watch the results take care of themselves.

50

Easy does it, but do it

Or: Why you should be the tortoise

In recovery, we have a saying, "Easy does it, but do it." I would say that everybody in recovery is behind the eight ball. Everybody is not up to speed in one or more areas of their life. It might be career, it might be relationships, it might be with your family. Everyone's deficient in some area when they first get into recovery; that's what it means to be unmanageable. What most people do is they start to rush to catch up. This is the worst thing you could do. Racing can make it worse.

What you have to do is slow down. This is what is meant by easy does it. If you get a good sponsor and he tells you to slow down, your normal tendency is to say, "Are you crazy?" But slow down is exactly what you have to do if you are going to win. Remember the race between the tortoise and the hare? Remember who won? It was the tortoise. Why? Remember, the tortoise was slow but steady. The hare, although fast, was inconsistent. So what happened was the tortoise won the race.

The Chinese have a saying, "Don't worry about making slow progress. Worry about making no progress."

Slow steady efforts, done over the long haul, will easily beat out large efforts done over a short period of time, then dropped. The sponsor I had before Carl was a college professor, and he used to say, "Easy does it. 'Does' is a verb – it doesn't say take it easy."

It's kind of like the great Oklahoma land rush of 1890. Everybody is on the starting line with horses, bicycles, motor-driven carts, and here you are walking. And then the bell goes off and there is a stampede. You want to race with everybody but your sponsor tells you to hold back, "easy does it." You say, "Are you nuts? I'm already behind. I'm on foot." He says, "Wait." This is to allow you to get a good footing. You start slowly, convinced you have lost the race. But as you proceed, you see the motorized car broken down along the side. One of the horses went lame. A wheel fell off a wagon. Well, you get the idea. The Bible says the last shall be first, and the first shall be last. It's almost as if the Good Book was talking about alcoholics. Close, but what I do think the Good Book was really talking about were people who had fallen off the path spiritually. That's you and me.

Here is another quote for you, and I believe this is from the Bible, too. "He who is master over small things, little things, will one day be master over great things and mighty things." Someone once asked me if I thought that statement was true. I said yes, largely because it says "master." Most people don't want to master anything anymore.

Start out on the path. Don't worry about people being ahead of you. Attend to your own path, your own footsteps, and in time you just might see all those motorized carts and wagon wheels left on the side of the road while you're still going for the finish.

GOOD LUCK.

ABOUT THE AUTHOR

Barry Bocchieri, MA, CADC, has practiced over sixteen years as a master's level certified addictions counselor. He began his own personal recovery over eighteen years ago. Everything he writes about in this book he has lived.

An expert in the field of substance abuse and addiction, he conducts seminars and workshops that are universally well received. It has been said that he has the unique ability of explaining complex psychological, philosophical, and spiritual concepts in clear, concise, and easy-to-understand language.

Barry Bocchieri is available for keynote speeches, as well as half-day and full-day seminars. Please address all inquiries to the author care of Idyll Arbor, 39129 264th Ave SE, Enumclaw, WA 98022, phone him at 732-572-9436, or e-mail tp AJMRBB@aol.com.

www.ingramcontent.com/pod-product-compliance
Lightning Source LLC
Chambersburg PA
CBHW072101040426
42334CB00041B/1824
9781882883660